The Women's Pill Book

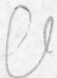

The **Women's** Pill Book

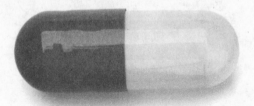

**Your Complete Guide
to Prescription and
Over-the-Counter
Medications**

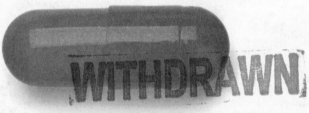

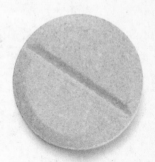

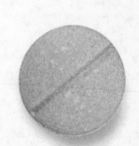

Deborah Mitchell

Consulting Medical Editor:
Marjorie Luckey, M.D.
*Associate Professor of Reproductive Science,
Mount Sinai Medical Center*

A Lynn Sonberg Book
St. Martin's Griffin ✿ New York

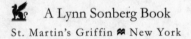

The information in this book is not intended to replace the advice of the reader's own physician or other medical professional. You should consult a medical professional in matters relating to health, especially if you have existing medical conditions, and before starting, stopping, or changing the dose of any medication you are taking. Individual readers are solely responsible for their own health-care decisions. The author and the publisher do not accept responsibility for any adverse effects individuals may claim to experience, whether directly or indirectly, from the information contained in this book.

The fact that an organization or Web site is mentioned in the book as a potential source of information does not mean that the author or the publisher endorse any of the information it may provide or recommendations it may make.

The stories in this book are composite, fictional accounts based on the experiences of many individuals. Similarities to any real person or persons are coincidental and unintentional.

THE WOMEN'S PILL BOOK. Copyright © 2012 by Lynn Sonberg. All rights reserved. Printed in the United States of America. For information, address St. Martin's Press, 175 Fifth Avenue, New York, N.Y. 10010.

www.stmartins.com

Design by Patrice Sheridan

ISBN 978-0-312-60382-3

First Edition: April 2012

10 9 8 7 6 5 4 3 2 1

Contents

Part Two: Drug and Supplement Profiles 67

Acknowledgments

The Women's Pill Book would not have been possible without the generous and skillful contributions of many people. I would like to thank Lynn Sonberg for conceiving the idea in the first place, and Dan Weiss and Meredith Mennitt at St. Martin's Press for recognizing that there was a need for this book in the marketplace. Special thanks are due to Marjorie Luckey, M.D., the consulting medical editor, for reviewing the narrative chapters of the book and making valuable suggestions. Finally, I acknowledge Antonio Carlos Jobim, my cat, who is as big as his name, for spending endless hours at my feet while I did the research necessary for this book. Needless to say, I remain responsible for any errors of fact or gaps in information in those chapters or in the pill profile portion of the book.

Introduction

Chances are, you picked up this book because you are a concerned, proactive woman when it comes to health. Most likely you spend time and energy taking care of your children's health, your partner's, and perhaps your parents' as well as your own health-care needs.

Overall, women are the largest consumers of medications, both over-the-counter (OTC) and prescription, and also the largest consumers of medical care. According to the National Center for Health Statistics Data Brief of September 2010, women are more likely (53.3%) than men (43.2%) to use prescription drugs.

But how much do you really know about the drugs your doctors are telling you to take? Even more important, how much information about prescription and OTC drugs is specifically targeted for women and your unique health-care needs?

The Women's Pill Book provides a complete and comprehensive guide to the medications women are being prescribed and taking for their health challenges, issues that are often completely different from those experienced by men.

Until now, women have had to make do with prescription and OTC pill guides that address either the entire population or adults in general. Darlene, a 52-year-old computer analyst, expressed frustration at the lack of drug information targeted for women. "I want a source that has information about drugs that are typically prescribed for health problems that solely or often affect women, like osteoporosis, menopause, migraines, fibromyalgia, and fatigue. And I want a source that provides information about the safety and side effects of those drugs."

Peggy, a 35-year-old mother of two, voiced similar sentiments. "I have fibromyalgia, and because of that I am prone to autoimmune diseases. I can't begin to tell you how many different drugs different doctors have recommended I take. It would be great to have a source that can help me understand my drug choices better and what to expect."

This book was designed with women like Darlene and Peggy in mind, plus every other woman who has ever wondered whether a certain prescription or OTC drug was safe to take, how it would affect her because she is pregnant or breast-feeding or going through menopause, which drugs she should be aware of if she is fighting chronic pain or is suffering with a chronic autoimmune disorder, and what is available for helping prevent heart disease.

Over the past decade, the percentage of Americans who took at least one prescription drug during the past month rose from 44% to 48%, while the use of two or more drugs increased from 25% to 31%. The most commonly used prescription drugs among adults ages 20–59 are antidepressants, painkillers, and cholesterol-lowering medications, and women make up the majority of users of these drugs. Among adults 60 years and older, cholesterol-lowering drugs, beta-blockers, and diuretics (both for high blood pressure and heart disease) make up the top three most used prescriptions.

Women and men are not the same when it comes to which drugs they take and the conditions they take them for, as well as how their bodies respond to and utilize those drugs. To quote the U.S. General Accounting Office's *Report to Congressional Requesters on Women's Health:*

> Women metabolize some drugs differently if they are pregnant, lactating, pre- or postmenopausal, menstruating, or using oral contraceptives or hormone replacements. Women's generally smaller body weight compared to men can result in higher levels of drug concentration in the blood stream. These and other established physiological and anatomical differences may make women differentially more susceptible to some drug-related health risks and demonstrate the importance of including women in all stages of drug development.

The report goes on to note that:

> In 1994, the Institute of Medicine reported that the FDA guidance that discouraged the participation of women of childbearing potential in initial small-scale trials led to the widespread exclusion of women in later large-scale trials. In addition, analyses of published clinical drug trials for life-threatening conditions have concluded that many past clinical trials included few or no women, making it uncertain whether the studies' results applied to women.

How to Use This Book

This book is divided into two parts. Part one consists of six chapters that address health issues of special interest to women:

- Reproductive health
- Chronic pain
- Autoimmune disorders
- Heart disease
- Hormonal challenges
- Prescription drug abuse

Each chapter provides the most up-to-date information that may help you better cope with and understand these health challenges. New studies and research results are being released all the time, and they often contain critical information about new drug treatments or dictate changes to the use of existing medications, all of which can be difficult to digest. That's why the first five chapters include information about the drugs health-care professionals are prescribing and recommending to treat the symptoms of the health challenges that may be affecting you or another woman in your life. The last chapter on prescription drug abuse can help you better understand the medications that are part of this growing problem and how you can identify them and get help. In each chapter, medications and supplements that have an entry in part two are in **boldface.**

These six introductory chapters also serve as launching points, sending you on to part two, where you can get in-depth information about drugs your doctor prescribes for you, drugs you hear about on TV or read about in magazines or on the Internet, medications your friends are taking and talking about, or drugs that have piqued your interest. For example, if you have been diagnosed with rheumatoid arthritis, the chapter on autoimmune disorders will introduce you to the challenges associated with treating this disease and some of the drugs you can investigate in part two. Likewise, if your best friend is dealing with chronic pain and doesn't know which drugs she should consider, you can refer her to the chapter on chronic pain and a discussion of the drugs to treat it. It also is not unusual to see commercials on TV for prescription drugs and be left wanting much more information about the product. Part two of this book can help you learn more.

Part two is arranged in an easy-to-follow format: All of the drugs and supplements are listed in alphabetical order by generic name (e.g., etanercept for Enbrel; calcium) and each entry follows the same format: brand name; generic; principal uses; about this drug; how to use this drug; side effects; possible drug, supplement, and/or food interactions; tell your doctor; of special interest to women; and symptoms of overdose. That is, you will find information that will help you better understand your medication and to also formulate questions to ask your health-care providers about medication and possible alternatives.

Finally, before we launch into the heart of the book, here are some questions you should ask your doctor and pharmacist about any medication that is prescribed:

- How long will I need to take it?
- What are the most common side effects?
- What are the severe side effects?
- What are the consequences of long-term use?
- Is a generic available?
- Are there any drug-to-drug, food, and/or supplement interactions associated with the use of this drug?
- Is this drug safe if I am pregnant or planning to get pregnant?

The information in this book can answer all but the first question, because the answer is different for each individual patient. Although every attempt is made to ensure the answers to these questions are up-to-date, you should always ask your health-care providers the same questions, as well as engage in some research on your own.

The results of new research and new studies can significantly change how or why you take a certain medication. Who can forget the results of the Women's Health Initiative, in which the use of synthetic hormone therapy was linked to an increased risk of breast cancer, stroke, and venous thrombosis, and maybe even increase the risk of coronary heart disease? Remember when the FDA pulled the arthritis and pain relievers Vioxx (rofecoxib) and Bextra (valdecoxib) off the market? Thus, a little extra time spent investigating any medications you are taking is time well spent.

Part One

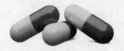

Health Challenges Facing
Today's Women

Chapter 1

Unique Reproductive Challenges

A woman's unique ability to become pregnant and give birth is a thing of joy and wonder, and a cause for celebration for women around the world. The underlying mechanisms involved in allowing birth to occur are extremely complex and encompass a myriad of intimately and intricately related elements. At the same time, there are numerous health issues that can affect a woman's ability to get pregnant, have a healthy pregnancy, and deliver a healthy child, including conditions such as abnormal menstrual function, polycystic ovarian syndrome, gynecologic cancers, endometriosis, pelvic inflammatory disease, and more.

In this chapter we look at the conditions and diseases that play a role in a woman's ability to get pregnant and give birth, the medications that are often prescribed to treat these health challenges, and how these medications may affect a woman's reproductive and overall health. (For your convenience, each medication entry in part two has a subheading titled "Of Special Interest to Women," where we note how a specific medication may affect a woman's reproductive health.) We also discuss the impact medications generally can have on a woman's health during pregnancy and after. These are times in a woman's life when her medication decisions affect not only her but her child as well.

Menstruation

Some women call it their period, others call it the curse. Perhaps you're at the stage in your life when you call it history! Whatever you call it, menstruation is central to a woman's reproductive health. Key elements of your reproductive health are hormones, and the hypothalamus and pituitary gland work together to control six of the main hormones necessary to keep your reproductive system functioning: estrogen, follicle-stimulating hormone (FSH), gonadotropin-releasing hormone (GnRH), luteinizing hormone (LH), progesterone, and testosterone.

This Is Your Period

Briefly, your menstrual cycle and these hormones work like this: Your hypothalamus releases GnRH, which triggers a chemical reaction in your pituitary gland to produce FSH and LH. In response to the release of FSH and LH, your ovaries produce estrogen, progesterone, and testosterone. The synchronization of all these hormones allows a normal menstrual cycle to occur.

Other substances involved with menstruation include prostaglandins, which cause your uterine muscles to contract so you can shed your menstrual blood. Women who have an excessive amount of prostaglandins in their uterus can experience very painful periods, a condition that is known as dysmenorrhea. Dysmenorrhea involves severe pelvic pain and often nausea and vomiting, back and thigh pain, headache, and other symptoms. An excess of prostaglandins is a cause of primary dysmenorrhea, while women who experience these symptoms as a side effect of other reproductive problems, such as endometriosis, pelvic inflammatory disease, uterine fibroids, or use of an IUD, are said to have secondary dysmenorrhea.

Treating Menstruation and Dysmenorrhea

If you still experience menstruation, chances are you also experience some annoying, uncomfortable, even distressing symptoms. While most women report mild to moderate symptoms of cramping, headache, breast tenderness, and bloating, others suffer more serious effects associated with dysmenorrhea. Statistics on how many women experience dysmenorrhea, range from 10% up to 90%, but the important thing is that if you are suffering with severe symptoms, the only statistic you care about is you, and you want relief.

For mild menstrual symptoms, a heating pad or a warm bath may be helpful. Some women report relief from natural remedies such as **black cohosh** or **fish oil,** and a limited number of scientific studies do back up their benefits. Effective over-the-counter or prescription nonsteroidal anti-inflammatory drugs (NSAIDs) such as **ibuprofen, mefenamic acid,** or naproxen can alleviate cramps and muscle aches, and are also helpful if you have dysmenorrhea, as these drugs reduce the concentrations of prostaglandins.

The FDA has approved the NSAIDs diclofenac, **ibuprofen,** ketoprofen, meclofenamate, **mefenamic acid,** and naproxen for treatment of dysmenorrhea. Your health-care provider may also prescribe oral contraceptives along with NSAIDs to treat your primary dysmenorrhea symptoms. If your doctor has determined that your severe menstrual symptoms are associated with another reproductive condition, it is necessary to treat that health issue simultaneously with your dysmenorrheal symptoms.

Menstruation Red Flags: See a Doctor If . . .

- Your period suddenly stops for more than 90 days (and you cannot attribute it to pregnancy or menopause).
- Your periods become very irregular after you have had regular cycles.
- Your period occurs more frequently than every 21 days or less often than every 45 days.
- You experience bleeding that is heavier than usual or you require one pad or tampon every 1–2 hours.
- You experience severe pain during your period.
- You bleed for more than 7 days.
- You experience fever and feel ill after using tampons.

Endometriosis

Between the start of menstruation and menopause, 10% of women can expect to experience endometriosis. If you are among this 10%, then you are likely no stranger to the pelvic pain that often—but not always—correlates to your menstrual cycle. For some women the pain occurs at other times of the month, and it can be so intense and debilitating that their lives are turned upside down for days.

What Is Endometriosis?

Endometriosis occurs when endometrial tissue, which should grow only inside the uterus, grows outside the uterus. These endometrial deposits, referred to as endometriomas, can be found on the ovaries, the fallopian tubes, the pelvic sidewall, the rectal-vaginal septum, and cesarean scars. Less often they are found on the appendix, bladder, bowel, colon, intestines, and rectum. Sometimes endometriosis causes adhesions that alter a woman's internal anatomy, and in advanced cases the internal organs can fuse together, causing what is known as a "frozen pelvis."

One of the more disturbing consequences of endometriosis for some women is an inability to have children. It is estimated that 30–40% of women with endometriosis suffer from infertility. If you are having difficulty getting pregnant and you have or suspect you have endometriosis, consult a knowledgeable physician as soon as possible to get a diagnosis. Although currently there is no cure for endometriosis, there are treatments that can significantly improve your quality of life.

Treatments for Endometriosis

Medication, hormones, nutritional therapy, alternative therapies, surgery— women have a variety of treatment options when faced with endometriosis. We focus on medications and hormones, but it is important to mention that some women respond to a holistic treatment approach that includes diet and lifestyle elements along with medical options, although these methods are less well studied.

Your choice of treatments will depend on your specific needs and your age, symptoms, and whether you have fertility issues. Many women rely on several treatment options over a long period of time.

Nonsteroidal anti-inflammatory drugs (e.g., **celecoxib, ibuprofen,** naproxen) are often used to treat endometriosis because they block the production of inflammatory substances called prostaglandins. Because women with endometriosis produce excess amounts of the prostaglandin PGE2, which causes inflammation, pain, and uterine contractions, NSAIDs can provide relief. However, because NSAIDs stop production of prostaglandins, these drugs must be taken before the prostaglandins are produced. That means you must begin taking the drugs at least 24 hours before you expect the pain to begin. If you wait until your pain starts, then the NSAIDs cannot stop the prostaglandins that have already been released into your system.

If you are taking NSAIDs to treat menstrual pain, it is recommended that you begin taking the medication at least 24 hours before you expect to start bleeding. If your crystal ball is not working and these events are unpredictable, you may want to begin taking NSAIDs about a week before you expect menstruation to begin. To prevent pain-producing prostaglandins from being released, you need to take the NSAIDs regularly as directed by your physician, typically every 6 hours around the clock. This is important because you want to block the release of any prostaglandins into your system. NSAIDs can also reduce the amount of menstrual bleeding. Important side effects and other information about the NSAIDs **celecoxib** and **ibuprofen** can be found in part two.

Other medications to relieve pain associated with endometriosis include **acetaminophen** (Tylenol) and narcotics (e.g., codeine, morphine). Unlike NSAIDs, these medications do not reduce prostaglandin synthesis, but they can help with existing pain.

Because estrogen stimulates the growth of endometrial tissue both inside and outside the uterus, hormone treatment can be prescribed to regulate estrogen production and inhibit the growth of endometrial lesions, and thus provide symptom relief. Your health-care provider may suggest combined oral contraceptive pills (estrogen plus progesterone) or progesterone/progestins alone. **Levonorgestrel** (Mirena), which has recently been shown to be effective for endometriosis and is used for this purpose in some countries, has not yet been approved in the United States for endometriosis. Because there are many different types of oral contraceptives and other hormone therapies, it is important that you discuss all the options and their benefits and risks with your health-care provider.

Another type of drug called GnRH (gonadotropin-releasing hormone) analogues has been used to treat endometriosis for more than two decades. Medications in this group include leuprolide and goserelin. Both are injected, and they dramatically lower estrogen levels and stop menstruation, which leads to shrinking and sometimes the disappearance of the endometriomas.

Endometriosis and Infertility

Generally, women who have endometriosis have more difficulty getting pregnant, but this does not mean it is impossible. Studies suggest that women who have mild endometriosis take longer to conceive, while those with moderate to severe disease have more difficulty. Some women turn to surgery or assisted reproductive technologies, or both, for help.

Gynecologic Cancers

Gynecologic cancers are those that affect a woman's reproductive tract and therefore the ability to conceive and give birth. The five main gynecologic cancers are cervical, ovarian, uterine, vaginal, and vulvar. A sixth type, fallopian tube cancer, is very rare. Four of the five main gynecologic cancers are typically diagnosed in women age 60 or older. Only cervical cancer is likely (47% of cases) to be diagnosed in women younger than 35. According to the Centers for Disease Control and Prevention (CDC), more than 80,000 women were given a diagnosis of a gynecologic cancer in 2007, and more than 27,000 women died from one of these types of cancer.

How can you help prevent gynecologic cancer or detect it early? Each of these gynecologic cancers has its own signs, symptoms, and risk factors, but there are some similarities as well. Perhaps most important is that if these cancers are detected early, treatment can be very effective. That's why it is critical for you to know your body and to seek medical attention if you recognize any warning signs of gynecologic cancers.

For example, the main cause of cervical, vaginal, and most vulvar cancers is human papillomavirus (HPV) infection, a common sexually transmitted virus. The HPV vaccine is available for women up through age 26 who did not get it at the age recommended by the CDC, which is 11–12 years old. You should also get a regular Pap test, which can detect precancerous changes on the cervix that can be treated so cervical cancer can be prevented. The Pap test does *not* detect any other type of gynecologic cancer.

Treatments for Gynecologic Cancers

Endometrial and cervical cancers, when identified early, are treated with surgery and/or radiation and do not require chemotherapy. More advanced cancers at these sites and other gynecologic cancers are typically treated using chemotherapy (drugs that stop or slow the growth of cancer cells), in addition to radiation therapy and/or surgery. The drugs chosen for treatment of gynecologic cancers depend on the type of cancer, stage of cancer, and your overall health. The drugs more often chosen as the "first-line" treatment—those health-care providers usually turn to first—include carboplatin (Paraplatin), **cisplatin** (Platinol), doxorubicin (Adriamycin), and paclitaxel (Taxol). Second-line treatments include 5-fluorouracil (Adrucil), **cyclophosphamide** (Cytoxan), etoposide (VePesid), and topotecan (Hycamtin).

Chemotherapy drugs are associated with bothersome side effects, and these are provided in the entries in part two.

Pelvic Inflammatory Disease

Every year, more than 750,000 women experience an episode of acute pelvic inflammatory disease (PID), an infection that affects the uterus, fallopian tubes, and other reproductive organs. The disease can damage the fallopian tubes and tissues in and adjacent to the ovaries and uterus, and lead to complications such as the development of abscesses, chronic pelvic pain, ectopic pregnancy, and infertility. In fact, more than 75,000 women may become infertile each year as a result of PID, and many ectopic pregnancies are associated with the disease.

How Do You Get PID?

Pelvic inflammatory disease is caused by bacteria that invade a woman's reproductive organs via the vagina and cervix. Although many different organisms can cause PID, a significant number of cases are associated with two very common sexually transmitted diseases—chlamydia and gonorrhea. Here's a quick look at both of these common causes of PID. (Read more about STDs under "Sexually Transmitted Diseases, Pregnancy, and Your Baby" below.)

According to the CDC, more than 1.2 million cases of chlamydia were reported in the United States in 2008, while the National Health and Nutrition Examination Survey estimated that nearly 3 million people age 14–39 were infected with *Chlamydia trachomatis*—the bacteria responsible for chlamydia and which can damage a woman's reproductive organs. About 10–15% of women with untreated chlamydia develop PID.

The danger associated with chlamydia is that although the symptoms (vaginal discharge, burning when urinating) may be mild or nonexistent, that does not stop the bacteria from causing serious and irreversible damage, including infertility, which can occur before women even know they have a problem. Women of childbearing age and who are sexually active are most at risk of contracting chlamydia and of developing PID. You increase your chances of getting PID the more sex partners you have, because there is greater potential for exposure to infectious organisms. You can also get re-infected if your sex partners are not treated.

Gonorrhea is caused by the bacteria *Neisseria gonorrhoeae*. The CDC esti-mates that more than 700,000 women and men in the United States get a new gonorrheal infection each year. Symptoms of gonorrhea are similar to those of chlamydia and also are typically mild or don't occur in women. Like chlamydia, the consequences of not treating this sexually transmitted disease can be serious.

Symptoms and Complications

As I've noted, it's easy to dismiss symptoms of PID. Along with an unusual vaginal discharge that may have a foul odor and painful urination, lower ab-dominal pain is common. Other symptoms include fever, painful intercourse, and irregular menstrual bleeding or spotting.

Because symptoms may be overlooked, women risk complications associ-ated with PID, including permanent damage to their reproductive organs. Scarring in your fallopian tubes and other structures in the pelvic area can cause chronic pelvic pain. Even if the fallopian tubes are only partially blocked or damaged, it can result in infertility. A damaged fallopian tube may also trap a fertilized egg in your tube. If the fertilized egg develops into an embryo in the tube rather than the uterus, it is called an ectopic pregnancy, a condition that can rupture the fallopian tube, causing severe pain, internal bleeding, and death.

Treatment of PID

The good news is that PID can be cured using antibiotics. The less than good news is that if any damage has already occurred, the antibiotics cannot reverse it. Therefore, if you experience pelvic pain or other symptoms of PID, seek medical care immediately. The sooner you treat PID, the better able you will be to prevent severe damage to your reproductive organs. Delaying treat-ment can result in infertility, the possibility of ectopic pregnancy, and chronic pelvic pain.

PID can be a challenge to treat because often more than one organism is responsible for the infection. That's why health-care providers often prescribe at least two antibiotics to address a wide range of possible culprits. The CDS no longer recommends antibiotics in the fluoroquinolone category for treatment of PID and gonococcal infections. Instead your doctor may prescribe **cephalexin** (Keflex) or cefotetan (Cefotan) (cephalosporin antibiotics) plus doxycycline (Doryx); clindamycin (Cleocin) plus gentamicin (Garamycin); or ampicillin and sulbactam (Unasyn) plus doxycycline (Doryx). You may also take an NSAID to help relieve pain or discomfort.

Occasionally, women with PID need to be hospitalized if they are severely ill with a high fever and vomiting, are pregnant, have an abscess in the fallopian tube or ovary, or are not responding to other treatments and need intravenous antibiotics. Surgery is rarely necessary.

Polycystic Ovarian Syndrome

About 6 million women in the United States have polycystic ovarian syndrome (PCOS), a condition in which a woman's hormones are out of balance because the ovaries make more androgens (male hormones, like testosterone) than normal. An imbalance of hormones can not only throw your periods out of whack, it can also make it very difficult to get pregnant, cause you to gain weight, contribute to skin problems, and eventually lead to serious problems such as heart disease and diabetes if it is not treated. Women with PCOS are also at an increased risk of uterine cancer.

Polycystic ovarian syndrome gets its name from the fact that most (but not all) women with the syndrome have small cysts on their ovaries. These cysts are follicles (eggs encased in a sac) that were never released during ovulation and remained in the ovaries. Women who have PCOS may have regular periods, but they may not ovulate (anovulatory cycles), which renders them unable to get pregnant.

Although these cysts are not harmful per se, they are the result of and contribute to hormone imbalances. Problems with the thyroid gland or other glandular problems can cause or contribute to a hormone imbalance as well.

Causes and Risk Factors

Even though PCOS is the most common hormonal syndrome affecting women of childbearing age in the world, the causes are not certain. It is likely there is more than one cause, and several possibilities are being considered by researchers:

- Dysfunction in the ovaries' production of testosterone and other male hormones
- A defect in the hypothalamus that causes excessive luteinizing hormone signals that stimulate the ovaries
- High levels of insulin, the result of insulin resistance, which increases the impact of luteinizing hormone on the ovaries
- Genetics—there is some evidence that PCOS may run in families

Symptoms of PCOS

PCOS is a syndrome and not disease, because it is a combination of various symptoms that all share an underlying cause. Some women experience many symptoms while others have only a few, and the severity of each symptom among women varies as well.

Basically, if you have PCOS, the production of testosterone and estrogen are out of balance. This may cause:

- Irregular periods or a lack of periods
- Appearance of facial and/or body hair
- Thinning hair on the scalp
- Acne
- Depression
- Insulin resistance, which can cause blood sugar levels to rise and eventually result in diabetes
- Abnormal blood lipid levels
- Weight gain and/or an inability to lose weight
- Infertility
- Darkening of the skin, especially at the nape of the neck
- Less common symptoms include white/gray breast discharge, pelvic pain, and/or development of skin tags

Treating Polycystic Ovarian Syndrome

Aside from medication, which we discuss below, dietary and lifestyle changes can help alleviate PCOS symptoms. Most women who have PCOS are also overweight, and weight loss with a healthy diet can not only help resolve symptoms by getting hormones back into balance, it can also reduce the risk of diabetes and heart problems. It is recommended that you seek a dietician who has experience working with women who have PCOS who can help you develop an effective eating program. Other steps you can take include regular exercise and stopping smoking, both of which can help reduce the risk of heart problems.

Medications used to treat PCOS include birth controls pills, **spironolactone,** and **metformin** (a diabetes medication). If you are trying to get pregnant, your health-care provider may recommend fertility medications.

Sexually Transmitted Diseases, Pregnancy, and Your Baby

Some sexually transmitted diseases (STDs) can cause infertility, as we saw with chlamydia, gonorrhea, and PID. However, STDs can also have a serious, even fatal, effect on your baby if you have one of these infections when you are pregnant. The good news is that bacterial STD, such as bacterial vaginosis, chlamydia, gonorrhea, and syphilis, can be treated and cured with antibiotics without affecting the fetus. STDs caused by a virus, however, such as HIV and genital herpes, can be treated to help reduce the risk of transmitting the virus to the fetus, but the disease cannot be cured.

Here's a look at some common STDs, how they can affect you and your fetus during pregnancy, and how they can be treated. As a precaution, women with an STD should ask their doctor about testing their partner for the disease, and whether they should use a condom or refrain from sex, including oral sex, and for how long.

Bacterial Vaginosis

Bacterial vaginosis is caused by an imbalance between the healthy and harmful bacteria in the vagina. Although controversial, it is thought that some women with bacterial vaginosis may develop PID as a result of the infection. Bacterial vaginosis increases susceptibility to other STDs, such as herpes simplex virus, chlamydia, and gonorrhea. If you have bacterial vaginosis while pregnant, you increase your risk for preterm delivery and for giving birth to an underweight infant. Bacterial vaginosis is treatable with antibiotics, most often clindamycin (Cleocin) or metronidazole (Flagyl).

Chlamydia

If you are pregnant and have chlamydia, the infection can be easily treated and cured with antibiotics, typically a single dose of **azithromycin.** Tetracyclines like doxycycline are contraindicated because they may cause staining of the developing child's teeth. If your sex partner has not been treated appropriately, you are still at high risk for re-infection. Left untreated, chlamydial infections may cause premature delivery. Chlamydia also is a significant cause of early infant pneumonia and pinkeye in newborns.

Gonorrhea

A pregnant woman can transmit the infection as her baby passes through the birth canal. This can cause blindness, joint infection, or a life-threatening blood infection in the baby. If you have gonorrhea and are pregnant, see your health-care provider immediately for treatment with an antibiotic to help minimize the risk of these complications.

Genital Herpes

About 1,500 newborns are affected by their mother's genital herpes each year in the United States, and this disease can be very serious for infants. The disease can be transmitted during delivery if you have active herpes; that is, if you are "shedding virus" at the time of delivery. You and your physician should discuss the possibility of a cesarean section to avoid exposing your infant to the virus.

If you learn you have genital herpes while you are pregnant, seek immediate medical treatment, which includes an antiviral medication such as **acyclovir** (Zovirax) or valacyclovir (Valtrex). Treatment during pregnancy can help reduce the risks to your child. About one-third of children infected with herpes at birth develop skin, eye, or mouth sores that can be resolved in nearly all cases with antiviral treatment. The central nervous system is affected in one-third of infants, who may develop symptoms such as seizures, fever, lethargy, and poor feeding behaviors. The remaining third develop disseminated herpes, which affects multiple organs. Genital herpes that affects the central nervous system and organs (e.g., liver, lungs) in infants can be very serious, and even with immediate treatment some die. Others can end up with serious long-term health problems.

HIV/AIDS

Human immunodeficiency virus (HIV) causes acquired immunodeficiency syndrome (AIDS). You can be HIV positive and not have AIDS. For most women who have HIV, the virus will not pass to the fetus if they are otherwise healthy, because the placenta provides protection. The infection may cross over, however, in women who have advanced HIV, malnutrition, an in-uterine infection (including an STD), or in those who recently acquired HIV.

Babies can become infected with HIV while in the womb, during delivery, or while breast-feeding. If you are pregnant and have HIV and are not being treated, there is a 25% chance your baby will be infected. With treatment, you can reduce that figure to less than 2%, according to the March of Dimes. The main type of treatment for HIV is antiretrovirals, of which there are about 20 in the United States, including amprenavir (Agenerase), efavirenz (Sustiva), and zidovudine (Retrovir).

Syphilis

Syphilis is an STD that is nearly nonexistent in childbearing heterosexual women in the United States, but some cases still exist. Fortunately, it is easy to cure: A single injection of penicillin can eliminate the disease if you have had syphilis for less than a year. If you are allergic to penicillin, your healthcare provider can treat you with other antibiotics. Getting treatment is critical, because the bacteria responsible for syphilis can infect the fetus during pregnancy. Depending on how long you have been infected, you may be at high risk of having a stillbirth or giving birth to an infant who dies shortly after birth. An infant may be infected yet have no signs or symptoms of the disease. If the infant is not treated immediately, however, he or she may develop serious problems such as seizures, or die.

Uterine Fibroids

Uterine fibroids are noncancerous growths that appear in or on the uterus in up to 75% of women of childbearing age. Most women are not even aware they have fibroids because in most cases these growths are problem-free, cause no symptoms, and require no treatment. Often they are discovered incidentally during a prenatal ultrasound or a pelvic exam.

In a small minority of women, however, uterine fibroids can cause pelvic pain, increased uterine bleeding, and infertility. Although most fibroids are microscopic or small, some can press on the fallopian tubes and block the passage of sperm or eggs, while others may distort the uterine wall and make it difficult for an egg to implant.

When uterine fibroids are problematic, treatment may include gonadotropin-releasing hormone agonists, such as leuprolide (Lupron), or androgens (male hormones), such as danazol, a synthetic drug similar to testosterone. These drugs can stop menstruation and shrink fibroids. NSAIDs can relieve pain, but they do nothing to shrink the fibroids or reduce bleeding.

If medication does not adequately resolve symptoms or if you and your health-care provider decide that removing the fibroids is necessary, especially if infertility is an issue, there are several surgical techniques that can be used, including uterine artery embolization and myomectomy, and an outpatient procedure called a hysteroscopic resection.

Other Reproductive Challenges

In addition to the conditions discussed already, there are a few other reproductive challenges women face. If you are attempting to get pregnant and are having difficulties, or you are experiencing problems with your periods, some of these factors may be involved:

- Overweight. Estrogen is stored in fat cells and tissues, and an excess of body fat can alter a woman's reproductive cycle.
- Underweight. Women whose body weight is 10–15% lower than normal may experience a lack of menstruation (amenorrhea).
- Use of medications. Some medications, including steroids such as cortisone and prednisone, which are used to treat lupus and asthma, can hinder production of follicle-stimulating hormone and luteinizing hormone and have a negative impact on ovulation if taken at high doses. Older blood pressure medications, such as Aldomet and Largactil, can raise prolactin levels and interfere with ovulation. Thyroid medications also can have an impact on ovulation if dosing is too high or too low. Drugs that affect the central nervous system, such as tranquilizers and anticonvulsives (e.g., valproic acid), can affect prolactin levels and impact menstruation.
- Autoimmune disorder. Problems with infertility can be a complication of some autoimmune disorders, such as diabetes, lupus, rheuma-

toid arthritis, and thyroid disease (an overactive or underactive thyroid gland).

- Tobacco and alcohol. Smoking may increase the risk of infertility, and as few as one drink per day can interfere with conception in some women.
- Environmental factors. Chronic exposure to high emotional or mental stress, radiation, chemicals (at home and/or at work and in everyday products such as plastics), and food additives and contaminants (e.g., bisphenol A [BPA]) may have an impact on fertility.

Chapter 2

Chronic Pain Challenges

As a mother, you may have asked your child to "tell me where it hurts." As a woman, you may have been asked the same question by your doctor or other health-care provider—or at least wish someone would ask. That's because women are much more likely to develop conditions characterized by chronic pain. Even the statistics are painful.

- Rheumatoid arthritis is 2–3 times more likely to develop in women, and women are also more likely to experience more severe symptoms than men.
- Women are 4 times more likely to have temporomandibular joint (TMJ) syndrome.
- Between 70% and 80% of cases of fibromyalgia—which is characterized by chronic pain—occur in women.
- Both tension and migraine headaches are more common in women, with migraines affecting 3 times more women than men.

Researchers report (and plenty of women will back them up!) that men and women experience pain differently, and that women experience chronic pain more frequently, with more intensity, and of longer duration. Women are also more likely to experience several painful conditions at the same time that compound both the physical and psychological pain, resulting in increased stress. The pain then becomes a vicious cycle that is a challenge to treat and defeat.

In this chapter we explore the challenges that women who live with chronic pain conditions face and the medications that are typically prescribed to treat them.

What Is Chronic Pain?

Chronic pain is defined as pain that lasts 6 months or longer without relief from treatment, whether medication, physical therapy, or psychological therapy. The pain can be associated with conditions such as fibromyalgia, migraine, rheumatoid arthritis, chronic fatigue syndrome, irritable bowel syndrome, among others. Do you or anyone you know have any of these conditions? Chances are very high that you do, and it's also a near certainty that those individuals are women, because all of these chronic pain disorders affect women more than they do men.

According to the International Association for the Study of Pain (IASP), "Chronic pain affects a higher proportion of women than men around the world, but unfortunately women are also less likely to receive treatment compared to men." The IASP attributes this lack of care to societal and cultural factors as well as economic barriers. The IASP felt so strongly about the issue of chronic pain in women that it announced a campaign called Real Women, Real Pain to draw attention to the impact chronic pain has on women.

If you live with chronic pain, you know the pain is real. If your health-care provider is unable to help you, it is time to find a new provider, research treatment options you have not considered before, contact support groups, and find someone who will support you in your quest for answers—a friend, family member, partner, or health-care worker. The mere act of taking control of your situation can alleviate some of the stress and make you feel empowered, which can in turn relieve some of the pain.

Pain and Hormones

How often do you blame how you feel on your hormones? If that thought crosses your mind often, you are not alone. In fact, it is on the minds of scientists as well, and they are dedicating quite a bit of research to the role of hormones in various illnesses that mostly affect women.

Take rheumatoid arthritis, for example. This painful autoimmune disease is more prevalent among women, suggesting a significant role for estrogen. Numerous studies have shown that estrogen has a role in migraine as well. Although sex hormones do not explain the difference between the sexes entirely, some connection is clear. First, women often experience their first migraine around the onset of menstruation in their teens. Most women who have migraines see a significant reduction or elimination of the pain during or after menopause, when estrogen levels drop dramatically.

Perception of pain seems to fluctuate with hormone changes as well. Some studies, for example, show that temporomandibular jaw pain is most intense when a woman is premenstrual or menstruating.

Emotions and Pain

The psychological aspect of pain is also critical. Generally, men focus on the physical sensations associated with pain while women may actually experience more intense pain because they focus on the emotional aspects and worry about how the pain will affect their lives and responsibilities.

Emotions can also be strong modulators of pain sensitivity. Researchers in the Netherlands evaluated clinical pain reports and pain sensitivity and threshold in response to strong emotions in women with and without fibromyalgia, and they got a surprise. Going into the study, they believed that negative emotions such as sadness and anger would increase pain in women who suffered with fibromyalgia but not in women without the disease. They found, however, that these emotions increased reports of pain and decreased pain threshold and pain tolerance in both groups of women. Anger and sadness appear to be general risk factors for amplification of pain. The greater the emotional response, the greater the pain.

One of the researchers, Henriët van Middendorp, PhD, of Utrecht University, pointed out that because "negative emotions are an unavoidable part of life, especially when you are dealing with chronic pain, it could be worthwhile to focus on trying to change the way people deal with their emotions in order to try to change the impact that negative emotions have on pain." This sounds like good advice that could significantly reduce a woman's dependence on medication to relieve chronic pain. Although Middendorp did not name ways for people to deal with their emotions, women with chronic pain may want to try support groups, counseling, relaxation therapies, meditation, and many other options.

There is even some evidence that in people with chronic pain, neurons in certain areas of the brain keep firing too much, and this could lead to permanent damage. A 2008 study conducted at Northwestern University, for example, used functional magnetic resonance imaging to scan the brains of people suffering with chronic back pain. The researchers found that in these patients, the front region of the cortex remained highly active. According to study author Dante Chialvo, associate research professor of physiology, "We know when neurons fire too much they may change their connections with other neurons or even die, because they can't sustain high activity for so long." Thus, chronic pain can alter brain function and cause problems such as sleep disturbances, depression, anxiety, and difficulty making simple decisions.

Pain Is in Your Brain

We all know that men and women are different, and one of the differences starts in the brain. A series of research studies conducted over the last decade suggest that the basic structure of the brain and how it operates is different in men and women. The differences could explain why women are more likely than men to experience and to seek help for chronic pain.

For example, studies indicate that men have a pain-dampening circuit that links their brain to their spinal cord. When this circuit is triggered by pain, the body's natural painkillers called endorphins are released and they decrease the pain. Some studies indicate that this circuit does not release as many endorphins in some women. Ouch!

This discovery could affect how pain and illness are treated in women. In the majority of cases, however, what scientists know about the brain and pain comes from studies of male animals and male human volunteers. Unfortunately, even though women experience more chronic pain, researchers have neglected to include enough females in studies of pain and how to prevent and treat this chronic and often life-altering problem.

Pain may even have the ability to change the structure of the brain. A study published in *Pain* found that women who experience menstrual cramps have significant changes in their brain structure compared with women who do not suffer with cramps. Specifically, researchers found that women who experienced dysmenorrhea (painful menstruation) had abnormal decreases in regions of gray matter involved in pain transmission and higher-level sensory processing and increases in areas involved in pain modulation. The scientists also reported that abnormal changes in gray matter were present in the women with dysmenorrhea even when they were not experiencing pain.

So what is a woman to do? I suggest communicate, medicate, and motivate.

Communicate Your Pain

If you want to get the best care possible, you need to take matters into your own hands. That does not mean you have to handle your chronic pain alone—not at all—but that you set the wheels in motion to get others to help you help yourself. A big part of that motion is finding a health-care provider with whom you feel comfortable and who listens to you and re-spects your concerns. Here are some ways to effectively communicate your pain.

- Keep a daily diary or log of your diet, sleep patterns, work and recre-ational activities, and symptoms. This may help you and your health-care provider see patterns that can be beneficial in managing your pain.
- Keep on top of the research on chronic pain and your specific condi-tion. Take notes so you can discuss anything that may be helpful with your doctor.
- When making a doctor's appointment, let the scheduler know you want some extra time to discuss questions or concerns. You will likely get only a few minutes, so be prepared with your written questions and notes when you get there.
- Take notes during your doctor visits so you will have a record of what transpired as well as a reminder of what you may need to do.
- If you tend to get nervous or upset during a doctor visit, bring a good friend or family member with you for support.
- Make sure all your doctors know what all your doctors are prescribing. It is also wise to always use the same pharmacy.
- Be assertive yet respectful in following up with your doctor about any concerns that arise after and between visits. Many doctors use e-mail to communicate with their patients, but they are busy, so give them a reasonable amount of time to reply.

- Seek support from family, friends, and support groups both in person and online. It is important to be able to comfortably share your concerns with others and to find people who understand what it means to have chronic pain.

Medications for Chronic Pain

Although medications are not the only way to help control chronic pain—many complementary/alternative methods are effective—they are a major source of relief for many women. Both prescription and over-the-counter drugs can be used, and all have at least some side effects. Because of the nature of chronic pain, it can be tempting to overuse or abuse some painkillers (discussed in chapter 6). To best treat your chronic pain condition and avoid abuse problems, you should work closely with your health-care provider(s) when choosing medication and making changes in drugs and dosages.

When prescribing drugs to treat chronic pain, the safest route is to begin with medications that are associated with the fewest side effects, such as **acetaminophen** or NSAIDs such as **ibuprofen** or naproxen, which are available OTC and by prescription. These are usually recommended for mild to moderate pain and to reduce inflammation. You should not take NSAIDs for longer than 10 days without talking to your doctor.

Not all pain relievers work on the same type or cause of pain, nor do they work in the same way, so it is important to consult your doctor when choosing pain relievers for side effects and counterindications such as harmful interactions if taken with other drugs, supplements, or foods.

- Anticonvulsants. Drugs in this category can reduce pain that originates in the nerves (neuropathic pain). Examples include **gabapentin** (Neurontin), which helps with shingles; **pregabalin** (Lyrica), which is effective in treating diabetic neuropathy; carbamazepine (Tegretol), lamotrigine (Lamictal), and oxcarbazepine (Trileptal), which are prescribed to treat facial pain associated with trigeminal neuralgia.
- Antidepressants. Not all antidepressants reduce pain, but some tricyclics, such as **amitriptyline,** can. Another type of antidepressant, **duloxetine** (Cymbalta), has approval from the Food and Drug Administration (FDA) for treatment of pain associated with fibromyalgia and peripheral neuropathy.

- Corticosteroids. These drugs, which include **prednisone,** dexameth-asone, and cortisone, can reduce pain related to inflammation. Oral corticosteroids affect the entire body and also suppress the immune system, a combination that can cause significant side effects, includ-ing weight gain, acne, thinning of the skin, and easy bruising, along with an increased risk of developing infections and osteoporosis. These drugs should be used only for the treatment of certain inflam-matory conditions, such as rheumatoid arthritis, utilizing the lowest dose and shortest treatment time possible.
- Opioid analgesics. These drugs are prescribed to treat moderate to severe pain. Examples include morphine, **oxycodone** (OxyContin), **hydrocodone with acetaminophen** (Vicodin), and **acetamino-phen** with codeine (Tylenol with codeine).
- Topical pain relievers. Sometimes a topical pain killer can be helpful, such as a lidocaine patch (Lidoderm), or a natural substance found in chili peppers called capsaicin, which changes pain messages in the skin.

If you are taking painkillers, it is important to be aware of the possible dangers and complications associated with their use, especially if you are of childbearing age, are pregnant or breast-feeding, drink alcohol, or are taking any other medications (prescription or OTC) or supplements. You can learn more about medications for treating chronic pain by talking with knowl-edgeable medical professionals and exploring the drug entries in part two of this book.

Some things to remember about drug treatment for chronic pain:

- Take the lowest possible dose that provides relief, and gradually in-crease the dose (with your doctor's help) only when necessary.
- Some medications take several weeks to kick in, so you may need to be patient.
- Never take higher doses than what your health-care provider has prescribed for you.
- Some medications may lose their effectiveness over time when used daily. Talk to your doctor if this occurs; never change your dose to a higher one than what your health-care provider has prescribed for you.
- Learn all you can about all medications and supplements you take and ask questions!

Motivate: What Else Can You Do?

Chronic pain should not run your life: You should. Although living with chronic pain is a challenge, many women step up to that challenge in a variety of ways. Here are some tips.

- Take back control of your life. Pain is not a simple adversary, so you need to attack it with a variety of strategies. Typically, no one pill or procedure or herbal remedy will relieve all your symptoms, so do your research and try different approaches, both conventional and alternative. If you are not pleased with your doctor, find a new one.
- Pace yourself. As you know, being in pain drains your physical and mental energies. If you try to do too much when you are having a good day, you will likely pay for it later. Spread out your tasks or activities and don't be afraid to ask for assistance.
- Maintain your body. Chronic pain takes a huge toll on the immune system, so it's important to follow a nutritious diet, exercise regularly, get enough sleep, and practice stress reduction.
- Stay engaged with life. It's important to stay connected with other people and to participate in enjoyable activities. It is all too easy to slip into a funk and depression, which makes the pain worse.
- Appreciate each day. It may sound Pollyanna, but look for the goodness in life. Find something in each day to be thankful for, something that is beautiful or touches your heart.

A Precautionary Tale

Many narcotic pain medications are combined with acetaminophen, another milder pain reliever. In high doses, however, acetaminophen can cause liver damage, and patients taking pain medication can inadvertently take toxic doses.

In 2010, the list of the most often prescribed drugs in the United States was released by IMS Health, a company that tracks the sales of pharmaceuticals for drug companies. At the top of the list was the painkiller Vicodin, an addictive medication that is a combination of the narcotic **hydrocodone with acetaminophen.** The drug is dangerous because once patients develop a tolerance for it, they begin taking too much, and this can lead to liver failure. The majority of the 400 people who die each year because of acetaminophen poisoning misused Vicodin or similar drugs.

The FDA's Sandra Kwede recently stated that "overdose from prescription combination products containing acetaminophen account for nearly half of all cases of acetaminophen-related liver failure in the United States, many of which result in liver transplant or death." It is important when taking pain medication to be aware of the dose of acetaminophen in all medications that you are taking, including that contained in OTC pain and arthritis remedies as well as many cold and flu relievers. Don't exceed 4000 mg/day if you are otherwise healthy; if you drink more than 3 drinks of alcohol per day, limit intake to no more than 2000 mg/day. If you already have liver disease, intake of any aceptominophen may be off-limits.

Chronic pain is difficult to diagnose and treat, and often women are prescribed multiple medications. It is critical that you know about and understand all medications you are taking and that you work with your healthcare provider to monitor your medication use and find safer alternatives or complementary approaches, including nutritional and herbal remedies and mind/body therapies such as acupuncture and meditation to help you best control your pain and improve your quality of life.

Chapter 3

Autoimmune Disorder Challenges

It's a fact: If you are female, you are significantly more likely than a male to develop an autoimmune disorder (autoimmune disease). An autoimmune disorder is a condition in which the immune system attacks the body's own healthy cells, tissues, and/or organs. Therefore, rather than do the job it was designed to do, the immune system triggers diseases that can involve the nervous, endocrine, and gastrointestinal systems, as well as the skin, eyes, connective tissues, blood, and blood vessels.

Experts do not yet understand why autoimmune disorders occur, nor exactly why they are so much more common among girls and women. It is known, however, that women have enhanced immune systems when compared with men. This is a positive thing because it increases your resistance to many infections. On the downside, it also makes you more vulnerable to autoimmune diseases.

Because the cause of autoimmune disorders remains much of a mystery, treatment—including medications—can be a challenge for patients and health-care providers. In this chapter we take a look at the challenges that autoimmune disorders pose to women and some of the medications that can tackle them.

Autoimmune Disorders in Women

According to the American Autoimmune Related Diseases Association, autoimmunity is the underlying cause of more than 100 serious, chronic illnesses that affect an estimated 23.5 million people in the United States, and about 75% of them are women. For some specific autoimmune disorders, such as Sjögren's syndrome, which affects approximately 4 million people, women represent an even higher percentage of those with the condition—in this case, 90%. Others, like Crohn's disease and psoriasis, affect men and women about equally. Here's a brief breakdown of some autoimmune disorders and the ratio of women to men:

- Hashimoto's thyroiditis: 10 to 1
- Systemic lupus erythematous (SLE): 9 to 1
- Sjögren syndrome: 9 to 1
- Antiphospholipid syndrome (secondary): 9 to 1
- Autoimmune hepatitis: 8 to 1
- Graves' disease (thyroid): 7 to 1
- Scleroderma: 3 to 1
- Rheumatoid arthritis: 2.5 to 1
- Multiple sclerosis: 2 to 1
- Myasthenia gravis: 2 to 1

Different ethnic groups also are more susceptible to certain autoimmune disorders. For example, Hispanic, Asian, Native American, and African-American women are two to three times more likely to develop lupus than Caucasian women.

You, Doctors, and Autoimmune Disorders

A major problem when dealing with autoimmune disorders is that too many medical practitioners are not aware of the genetic predisposition. to develop them. If they were, they might be more likely to concentrate on getting a thorough family medical history from women who come to them with perplexing symptoms. There can be many clues in the symptoms, diseases, and ailments experienced by a woman's mother, father, siblings, and grandparents.

Another problem is that autoimmune disorders mostly affect younger women in their childbearing years. These women often look healthy, so doctors frequently do not take their symptoms seriously. One reason for this neglect is that symptoms often are vague at the beginning and difficult to describe accurately. Fatigue, pain, gastrointestinal problems, and overall aches and stiffness may develop gradually, come and go, or creep up on you. It is easy to discount these symptoms as being related to your period, working too hard, stress from your kids or your job, and then dismiss them until they become so persistent and life altering that you can't ignore them any longer.

You may be nodding your head and know exactly what I am saying. You may have experienced the frustrations of getting a diagnosis for your autoimmune condition and then the challenge of finding effective treatments. Some women go from doctor to doctor, spending months, even years, looking for answers to why they are experiencing the symptoms they do. That woman does not have to be you.

A study by the American Autoimmune Related Diseases Association found that more than 45% of people with autoimmune diseases had been called chronic complainers during the earliest stages of their disorders. Placing such a label on a young woman can ruin her life if she delays or stops seeking help for her symptoms.

Finding Information and Getting Professional Help

If you suspect you may have an autoimmune disorder and you have not been able to find a health-care professional who will work with you, then it is time to take steps.

- Educate yourself about your symptoms through research on the Internet by visiting reputable health Web sites (see Resources).
- Contact organizations that are dedicated to the condition or conditions you believe you have, such as the Arthritis Foundation, Lupus Foundation, etc. (see Resources). Such organizations provide not only information about the disorder but also typically the names of qualified practitioners in your area as well as support groups and/or forums (online and/or locations in your area).
- Visit and/or participate in support groups or forums to learn more about autoimmune conditions.

- Attend lectures, presentations, and health fairs given in the community or at health-care facilities by medical professionals. These can be an opportunity to meet and speak with knowledgeable individuals who may help you with your search.
- Keep a detailed journal of your symptoms, any treatments you try (including OTC and prescription medications, nutritional supplements, herbal remedies, any procedures or alternative therapies), and any relevant information you gather from your research and/or interaction with organizations and support groups.
- Look for clinical trials. Requirements to participate in a clinical trial vary greatly from one trial to another, so it is necessary to carefully read the requirements for each one. You can get detailed information about available clinical trials at http://clinicaltrials.gov.

The more information you have, the better able you will be to help your doctor diagnose your condition and participate in developing the best course of treatment that fits your needs and lifestyle.

Medications for Autoimmune Diseases

The category of autoimmune diseases and their symptoms is so broad that it is not possible to address all the different medications your health-care provider could prescribe. However, autoimmune diseases have one thing in common: The body's immune system overreacts, causing damage to cells, tissues, and/or organs. This core problem is treated with immunosuppressive drugs, which decrease the immune response. Although corticosteroids can also suppress the immune system (see chapter 2), drugs in the immunosuppressive category are much more powerful and can be safer for longer-term use.

Immunosuppressive drugs can act in different ways in the body: Some inhibit the activity of certain genes while others reduce inflammation or stop an allergic response. Although these drugs are often beneficial, they can take a serious toll on your health, and the reason is right in their name: They suppress the immune system and they do so indiscriminantly, suppressing both overly active responses and protective ones. This means you are at greater risk of developing infections and cancer if you are taking immunosuppressive medications. Not all immunosuppressive drugs carry the same level of risk for these serious problems, but they are a significant concern and something you need to discuss with your health-care provider. Here are some of the immunosuppressive drugs commonly prescribed for different autoimmune disorders.

- adalimumab (Humira): rheumatoid arthritis, psoriatic arthritis, ankylosing spondylitis, Crohn's disease
- anakinra (Kineret): rheumatoid arthritis
- **azathioprine** (Imuran): lupus, rheumatoid arthritis, chronic ulcerative colitis
- **cyclophosphamide** (Cytoxan): lupus, rheumatoid arthritis, scleroderma
- **cyclosporine** (Sandimmune): psoriasis, rheumatoid arthritis, multiple sclerosis, myasthenia gravis, diabetes
- **etanercept** (Enbrel): rheumatoid arthritis
- **glatiramer** (Copaxone): multiple sclerosis
- **infliximab** (Remicade): Crohn's disease, rheumatoid arthritis, psoriasis, ankylosing spondylitis, psoriatic arthritis
- IVIG (intravenous immunoglobulin, made from human plasma): rheumatoid arthritis, diabetes, multiple sclerosis, myasthenia gravis
- leflunomide (Arava): rheumatoid arthritis
- mercaptopurine (Purinethol): Crohn's disease, ulcerative colitis, psoriatic arthritis
- **methotrexate** (Trexall): psoriasis, rheumatoid arthritis
- rituximab (Rituxan): rheumatoid arthritis
- **sulfasalazine** (Azulfidine): ulcerative colitis, rheumatoid arthritis, Crohn's disease

NOTE: If you have an autoimmune disease and you plan to get pregnant or are pregnant, you and your doctor need to weigh the risks of harm to the fetus from use of any immunosuppressive medications against the need to control your disease during pregnancy and postpartum. This is an individual decision and the circumstances vary from woman to woman. In fact, the topic of medication use during pregnancy for women who have an autoimmune disorder is so important it deserves a closer look.

Autoimmune Disorders, Pregnancy, and Medications

Generally, women who have an autoimmune disease can get pregnant and have children without encountering any health challenges. In fact, symptoms of autoimmune thyroid diseases and some other autoimmune conditions tend to improve during pregnancy. However, the symptoms reappear after delivery. That said, certain autoimmune disorders are associated with more potential risks to the mother and/or child than others.

For example, pregnant women who have lupus have a greater risk of stillbirth, delivering a preterm infant due to preeclampsia, having a smaller than normal fetus, and recurrent spontaneous abortion. Unfortunately, the course of preexisting lupus during pregnancy is unpredictable, but symptoms may worsen, especially immediately postpartum. If you have severe lupus, you may need to continue taking immunosuppressant medications during your pregnancy (e.g., hydroxychloroquine). This is a decision you and your doctor will need to make after discussing the risks and benefits. (Also see "Medications for Autoimmune Diseases" above).

Rheumatoid arthritis can develop during pregnancy or, more frequently, begin after delivery. If you develop rheumatoid arthritis during pregnancy, the first choice of medication is usually **prednisone.** If you already have rheumatoid arthritis and become pregnant, chances are good your symptoms will improve during pregnancy. This autoimmune disorder does not usually have an impact on the fetus, but your delivery may be difficult if the arthritis affects your lumbar spine, pelvis, or hip joints.

Pregnant women who have myasthenia gravis frequently experience breathing difficulties during pregnancy, and they are also extremely sensitive to medications that suppress respiration, such as sedatives. Some women with myasthenia gravis require increasing doses of anticholinesterase drugs (e.g., **neostigmine**) or atropine during pregnancy, and you need to discuss the potential benefits and risks of such medications with your health-care provider.

Antiphospholipid syndrome (APS; also known as Hughes syndrome) is an autoimmune disorder in which the body produces large amounts of antiphospholipid antibodies. These antibodies attack the special fats (phospholipids) that make up the outer walls of all cells in the body. This disease often occurs along with lupus and other autoimmune disorders common in women.

Women with APS who are pregnant are at increased risk of stroke and blood clots. Other serious complications include a higher chance for pregnancy-induced hypertension (in up to 50% of women with the disorder), stillbirth, recurrent miscarriages, poor fetal growth, and preterm births, as well as cardiovascular disease.

Even though APS is a serious disease, most doctors do not check for it in patients who have an autoimmune disease, except possibly those who have lupus. Therefore, if you have an autoimmune condition and you plan to get pregnant or are pregnant, you should ask your health-care provider about the possibility of your having APS.

An estimated 0.3–0.5% of pregnant women have overt hypothyroidism, while subclinical hypothyroidism occurs in 2–3% and hyperthyroidism is seen in up to 0.4%. In addition, many medications may not be safe if they are taken during pregnancy, and this is an important issue discussed in every drug and supplement entry in part II of this book.

If you have an autoimmune disorder and you are having difficulty getting pregnant, talk to your doctor. He or she may suggest that you wait until your disease is in remission or that you change your medications before you start or continue trying to get pregnant. Also consider consulting a physician who is familiar with high-risk pregnancies. Your doctor may also suggest you undergo tests to determine if your fertility challenges are caused by an autoimmune disease or an unrelated reason.

What You Can Do to Help Yourself

If you have been diagnosed with a chronic autoimmune disorder, you may be experiencing a variety of feelings and asking yourself how you are going to learn to live with this life-altering condition. If you got the diagnosis recently, those emotions and questions may be heavy on your mind. If you have been living with the disorder for some time, you have likely found ways to cope with your symptoms. In either case, the following tips and guidelines can help you better manage your illness so that it does not manage you.

- Ask questions. Do not be afraid to ask your health-care provider(s) questions about your condition and your treatment, including any information you discover that your doctors have not addressed.
- Keep your doctor informed. If you develop any new symptoms or your current symptoms worsen, let your doctor know. Put aside any fear that your doctor may think you are a hypochondriac; your new symptoms may be an indication that something is wrong and needs to be addressed.
- Take all medications as directed by your health-care provider. Do not start, stop, or change any treatment program without first consulting your doctor.
- Pace yourself. One of the most common symptoms among autoimmune diseases is fatigue, and at times it can be debilitating. Therefore,

be aware that fatigue may be a life-altering factor for you and make plans to deal with it. You may need to schedule naps or rest periods, ask for help with certain tasks, and spread out your tasks over a longer time period. Learn to listen to your body and allocate your activities so you do not overburden yourself.

- Pay attention to your diet. It's easy to neglect your nutrition if you are overly tired, depressed, experiencing pain, or other chronic symptoms that are characteristic of many autoimmune disorders. However, poor dietary choices can exacerbate your symptoms. If sticking to a healthy diet is a challenge, ask your physician, a dietician, other health-care providers, or support group members for suggestions and help.

- Be prepared for emotionally exhausting days. Having a chronic autoimmune disease can be emotionally tiring as well as physically challenging. If you have days when your symptoms don't allow you to do the things you want to do, you may experience anger, fear, and depression, as well as feelings of isolation. If you understand that such feelings can happen, you can prepare for them by making a plan, such as having certain people you can call, joining a support group, practicing stress reduction techniques, or allowing yourself a special treat. At the very least, acknowledge that such feelings can occur and will pass.

Chapter 4

Heart Disease Challenges

When it comes to matters of the heart, women have some big challenges to face. No, I'm not talking about love! I'm talking about heart disease. The truth is, the majority of women are not even aware that they should be paying more attention to their heart. According to the Women's Heart Foundation, more than 60% of women believe breast cancer is their biggest health threat, but in fact heart disease kills six times as many women as breast cancer.

More specifically, heart disease is the number one killer of women. A sad and little known fact is that more women die from heart disease than men, according to the latest (2010) statistics from the American Heart Association. Heart disease is also the most common cause of female disability in the United States.

The encouraging news is that heart disease is largely a preventable condition. If you practice positive lifestyle habits and understand the warning signs of heart disease, you can significantly reduce your risk.

In this chapter we look at the challenge of heart disease in women: the warning signs, how to prevent heart disease, and some critical information about medications your health-care providers may prescribe that may affect your heart. Because it is common for women who have a heart condition to take more than one medication, it is important to know the possible side effects of those medications and any potential interactions between them and other drugs, supplements, or foods. More specific information about individual drugs your doctor may prescribe for you is covered in the drug and supplement entries in part two.

Now, let's take a look at your heart.

Women and Heart Disease

If you take nothing else away with you from this chapter, let it be this: Know the warning symptoms of a heart attack for women. The early warning signs of heart disease in women—and the symptoms during an actual heart attack—do not follow the classic patterns that men exhibit and are often ignored or misdiagnosed by health-care providers, especially in premenopausal women. That means women often not only miss the signs of an impending heart problem but may also have to maneuver their way through an uncooperative medical community to get lifesaving attention and care.

Case in point: A landmark study by the National Institutes of Health (NIH) titled "Women's Early Warning Symptoms of AMI" (acute myocardial infarction, or heart attack), published in *Circulation: Journal of the American Heart Institute* in 2009, reported that 95% of women who had experienced a heart attack said they had had symptoms in the weeks and months before their attack, but the symptoms did not include the "normal" symptom: chest pain. Therefore, they ignored their symptoms and did not recognize they were candidates for a heart attack—until it happened.

Symptoms of a Heart Attack

True or false? The most common symptom of heart attack among women is chest pain. If you said false, then you know something that could save your life. In fact, chest discomfort, often described as a tightness or heaviness in the center of the chest that may or may not radiate to other parts of the body, is the most common symptom of a heart attack in men. Among women, however, it is a different story.

In the NIH study, of the 515 women who had suffered a heart attack, less than one-third said they had had any chest pain or discomfort before the attack, and 43% said they had no chest pain during any phase of the attack. They did, however, report other symptoms, ones you may not normally think of when talking about a heart attack. Being attuned to these symptoms could save your life. So here they are.

- Fatigue or exhaustion. In the NIH study, more than 70% of women experienced extreme fatigue in the weeks or months before they had their heart attack. If you have significant fatigue that prevents you from doing your normal activities and it lasts for several days, this could be a symptom of heart trouble. It's time to call your doctor.

- Nausea or indigestion. This symptom of a heart attack is often ignored, and of course it is easy to see why. Who doesn't experience some stomach upset once in a while? However, you should be alert to anything unusual, especially if it occurs suddenly and you haven't eaten anything that should cause nausea, cramping, vomiting, or indigestion. Women and adults older than 60 are more likely to experience this symptom of a heart attack. In the NIH study, indigestion before the attack was reported by 39% of the women.

- Dizziness and shortness of breath. More than 40% of the women in the NIH study experienced breathlessness and dizziness before their attack, while 58% said they had it during the attack. If your heart is not able to get enough blood and oxygen, it may be unable to pump enough blood to the lungs or the brain, and you may then experience shortness of breath and light-headedness or dizziness. One reason people rarely associate these symptoms with a heart attack is that they think something is wrong with their lungs, not their heart.

- Anxiety and sleep problems. These two symptoms seem to go hand in hand. Many of the women in the NIH study felt a sense of "impending doom" in the weeks and months before their heart attack. Almost half said they had trouble sleeping and 35% reported anxiety. Of course, if you already have insomnia or other sleep problems, this symptom will likely go unnoticed. But if you do not usually have trouble sleeping or suffer with anxiety, then these could be notable indicators.

- Swelling or pain in the legs. If your heart is not functioning properly, blood flow to the kidneys is reduced and the pressure in the veins can increase, causing fluid to accumulate in your tissues, resulting in swelling or edema. Because your feet, ankles, and legs are farthest from your heart, swelling usually starts there. You should contact your doctor if you experience any swelling in your legs.

- Jaw, ear, shoulder, elbow, or neck pain. Rather than chest pain, many people who have a heart attack experience pain that runs along their jaw or near their ears, or in the shoulder and neck area. Some women report feeling pain between their shoulder blades and down into their elbows. This is another difficult symptom to pinpoint, but if you feel pain in any of these areas, you should contact your doctor.
- Rapid heart rate or pulse. The fancy name for this symptom is tachycardia. Such episodes typically come on suddenly and last only a few seconds, but if they last longer they can also cause sweats, dizziness, weakness, and sometimes loss of consciousness. Women often dismiss these events as panic attacks, but they may be a warning of a heart attack.

Medications and Heart Risks

It is important to stay current on information about medications and their possible impact on heart health. For example, phenylpropanolamine (PPA), an ingredient commonly included in OTC and prescription cold and cough medications and weight-loss products, was found to increase the risk of bleeding into the brain or tissue around the brain in women. (This same risk, however, was not found in men.) Fortunately, PPA has been removed from the market, but for many years women had unknowingly exposed themselves to this risk.

Some prescription medications, even if you take them as prescribed by your doctor, can have a detrimental effect on your heart. In rare cases they can even put you at risk for sudden cardiac death. One reason many drugs can impact even a healthy heart is that they alter the body's normal blood levels of certain minerals called electrolytes (magnesium, calcium, sodium, potassium), which are necessary in a proper balance to maintain normal heart function.

For example, diuretics (e.g., **furosemide, hydrochlorothiazide**), also known as water pills, which are commonly prescribed to treat high blood pressure, heart failure, and edema, cause an increase in urination and an accompanying reduction in the amount of fluid in the body. The problem is that the excess urine also carries an excessive amount of critical electrolytes out of the body. The result can be a range of symptoms, including abnormally low blood pressure, sleepiness, dizziness, dry mouth, rapid heartbeat, muscle pain and cramps, and confusion. For this reason, your doctor may recommend that you take mineral supplements to prevent low levels of electrolytes. However, if you have done your homework about a diuretic your doctor prescribes and you see that it may deplete your electrolytes, you can be proactive and ask him or her how to prevent this from happening.

Other medications for the heart can affect the blood vessels or the ability of the heart to pump blood. Beta-adrenergic blockers (beta-blockers), such as atenolol and **metoprolol,** are prescribed for high blood pressure or to reduce stress on the heart. They achieve this by slowing the heart rate and relaxing the arteries. In some people, however, beta-blockers can cause excessive slowing of the heart rhythm, especially if you already have a very slow heart rate. In rare cases, beta-blockers can contribute to heart failure by suppressing the heart's ability to pump blood.

ACE (angiotensin-converting enzyme) inhibitors are prescribed for high blood pressure and heart failure, and to help prevent stroke or heart attack if you are at risk. Drugs in this group include captopril, enalapril, and **lisinopril.** Drugs in this class rarely cause irregular heartbeat and an increase in potassium levels. Abnormally high potassium levels can cause weakness, tiredness, irregular heartbeat, and mild paralysis.

Antiarrhythmic drugs offer lifesaving benefits for many women who experience abnormal heart rhythms, and the advantages outweigh the risks. Infrequently, however, they may cause new heart rhythm problems or make existing ones worse, and in rare cases cause heart rhythm disorders that lead to sudden cardiac death. Discuss the benefits vs. risks with your doctor.

Supplements and Heart Risks

Since women are the largest users of nutritional and herbal supplements, you should be aware that combining some of these natural substances with OTC or prescription medication, including those for the heart, can cause some serious health problems. This is why it is critical that you *always* let your doctor know if you are taking any type of nutritional or herbal supplement before you begin a new medication. Nutritional and herbal supplements can be just as potent as or even more so than medications.

For example, Saint-John's-wort, which is used to treat depression and sleep disorders, has an effect on the liver, which is involved in the metabolism of most medications, especially those prescribed for the heart. Therefore, if you are using Saint-John's-wort and your doctor prescribes a heart medication, you need to talk to your doctor about this, because the herb can reduce the activity of blood pressure and rhythm-controlling medications.

Similarly, be cautious if you are taking any natural supplements that can increase your risk of bleeding, such as ginkgo biloba or garlic, if you are also prescribed a blood-thinning medication such as **warfarin.** Even some food and beverages can pose a risk if taken with heart medications. Grapefruit and grapefruit juice, for example, interfere with the enzymes that break down drugs such as statins, which are used to lower cholesterol, and amiodarone, which is used to treat abnormal heart rhythms. These are the types of warnings included in the drug entries in part II.

Hormone Replacement Therapy and Heart Risks

For many years, scientists believed that hormone replacement therapy (HRT) could reduce women's risk of heart disease at all ages. According to the results of large studies such as the Women's Health Initiative (WHI) and the Heart and Estrogen/Progestin Replacement Study (HERS), however, it appears that the story is more complicated and the effects on heart disease risk differ depending on whether women take estrogen alone or with medroxyprogesterone acetate (Provera). The timing of initiation of treatment is also an important factor.

In women who take estrogen alone (without Provera), the research showed a statistically significant reduction in the number of heart attacks, coronary deaths, and the need for cardiac surgery in women who started estrogen-only treatment during age 50–59. However, women who initiated either estrogen alone or estrogen with medroxyprogesterone acetate more than 10 years beyond the onset of menopause were found to be at increased risk for serious heart disease. Among women who initiated hormone therapy closer to menopause (within 10 years), the tendency was for a lower risk of coronary heart disease.

In addition, the results of HERS showed that continuous HRT in women who had coronary heart disease did not reduce their cardiovascular risk, and both HERS and WHI showed that oral estrogen increases the risk of thromboembolic events—the formation of a clot (thrombus) in a blood vessel, which can break away from the vessel and be carried to another part of the body, where it can block a vessel in the lungs, brain, kidneys, leg, or gastrointestinal tract.

As a result of these studies, while estrogen use continues to be indicated for the relief of significant menopausal symptoms, experts warn that HRT should not be used to reduce a woman's cardiovascular risk.

The bottom line: If you are considering HRT, you and your doctor need to have a serious discussion about the benefits and risks, especially if you have a heart condition. You can read more about hormones and the challenges they present to women in chapter 5.

Heart Disease: Are You at Risk?

Now that you are familiar with the symptoms of a heart attack, what do you know about your risks of heart disease? According to the National Coalition for Women with Heart Disease, an estimated 42 million American women live with some form of cardiovascular disease. Are you one of them? Are you at risk for a heart attack, angina, sudden cardiac death, or other heart conditions?

There are two groups of risk factors. One is the traditional risk factors for heart disease—high cholesterol, high blood pressure, obesity, and diabetes, which affect both women and men about equally. To know where you stand in terms of risk for heart disease in these areas, here are some of the "good" numbers you want to see on your test results.

- Total cholesterol: less than 200 mg/dL
- LDL (low-density lipoprotein) "bad" cholesterol:
  - optimal: less than 100 mg/dL
  - near optimal: 100–129 mg/dL
  - borderline high: 130–159 mg/dL
  - high: 160–189 mg/dL
  - very high: 190+ mg/dL
- HDL (high-density lipoprotein) "good" cholesterol: 50+ mg/dL
- Triglycerides (a type of fat found in the blood): less than 150 mg/dL
- Blood pressure: less than 120/80 mmHg
- Fasting glucose level: less than 100 mg/dL
- Body mass index (BMI): less than 25
- Waist circumference: less than 35 inches

Other factors that may have a larger role in the development of heart disease in women:

- Depression and mental stress.
- Smoking cigarettes increases your risk of dying from heart disease by 2–3 times.

- Metabolic syndrome—a combination of high blood pressure, high blood sugar, high triglycerides, and excess fat around your abdomen.
- Low levels of estrogen after menopause place women at a significant risk for developing cardiovascular disease in the smaller blood vessels.
- Lack of exercise is a risk factor for heart disease, and many women are not getting the physical activity they need. Half of Caucasian women, 64% of African-American women, 60% of Hispanic women, and 53% of Asian/Pacific Island women are sedentary.
- Women who have diabetes are 2.5 times more likely to have a heart attack than women without diabetes.

Helping Yourself Avoid Heart Disease

When you consider all these facts and statistics together, the picture is not a rosy one. The question is: What are you going to do to make sure you are not one of these statistics? We all know that even the best intentions can go awry, and following a heart-healthy lifestyle can be a road littered with hurdles. Job stressors, love relationships, raising children, financial problems, social obligations, aging parents—the list of things that can keep you from taking care of yourself and your heart can be overwhelming at times.

However, you are worth the effort. I hope your answer to the question includes the following, especially if you are menopausal, as the dramatic decline in estrogen that accompanies menopause raises your risk of heart disease.

- Follow a diet low in saturated fat (less than 7% daily intake) and trans fat (partially hydrogenated fats such as shortening and margarine; also found in fast food and snack foods).
- Adopt a high-fiber diet, with 25–30 grams of fiber daily, which can be found in whole grains, legumes, fruits, and vegetables.
- Participate in aerobic exercise for at least 30–40 minutes 4–5 times a week.
- Reduce stress: High levels of stress hormones are a great strain on the heart.
- Do not smoke.
- Get 7–8 hours of sleep per night.
- Treat medical conditions such as diabetes, high blood pressure, obesity, and high cholesterol, all of which are known risk factors for heart disease.
- Socialize often.

- Become familiar with all medications (OTC and prescription) as well as supplements you plan to take, including possible interactions, side effects, and precautions.

Another word of advice as you take steps to protect yourself against heart disease: Be assertive when dealing with the medical community. According to the American Heart Association Statistics Committee and Stroke Statistics Subcommittee (2010), women are less likely than men to receive appropriate treatment after experiencing a heart attack, a fact that may have a direct bearing on the following statistics: 23% of women and 18% of men die within 1 year of a first recognized heart attack, and 22–32% of women and 15–27% of men heart attack survivors will die within 5 years.

In a study released in 2011 by the University of Michigan Cardiovascular Center, the researchers reported that although women overall have a higher in-hospital death rate from a severe heart attack, the difference is related to a woman's age and any additional health problems she has, not gender specifically. For example, although women make up only about one-third of patients who undergo cardiac procedures, they tend to be older and to have more comorbidities (additional health problems) along with their heart disease. Women are also more likely to experience vascular complications or hemorrhaging in the hospital that requires a transfusion. All of these factors increase the rate of in-hospital deaths from heart attack.

Two more disturbing statistics that will, I hope, prompt you to take better care of your heart and yourself. One is that women make up only 27% of participants in all heart-related research studies, according to a study published in the *Journal of Women's Health* (June 2003). Although this percentage has (hopefully) risen since this statistic was released, it is still a grim reminder that there is likely much experts do not know about how women respond to heart-related medications. This means you need to be even more proactive and vigilant about your medication use.

The American Heart Association released some troubling information. It noted that in 2006, about 79% of women who were experiencing signs of a heart attack said they would call 911. But by 2009, that number had declined to 50%. Don't be your own worst enemy! Yes, the signs of a heart attack can be misleading, but if you think you are having a heart attack, get immediate medical attention.

Take charge of your heart health!

Chapter 5

Hormonal Challenges

Beyond the impact that your hormones have on menstruation, pregnancy, and menopause, they have a unique influence on other aspects of your health. Osteoporosis in women, for example, is caused, at least in part, by the decline in estrogen levels, especially at the time of menopause. Eighty percent of osteoporosis cases are in women. Hormones are believed to have a role in depression as well, and the mood swings associated with menopause and PMS are well documented. Furthermore, a woman's estrogen levels may influence her risk of developing Alzheimer's disease. Hormones are indeed a challenge in your life, affecting you from your head to your toes, but one that can be managed.

In this chapter we look at the role of hormones in a number of health challenges women face and the medications your health-care providers may prescribe to treat them.

Alzheimer's Disease and Other Dementias

What role do hormones have in Alzheimer's disease and other types of dementia? The Women's Health Initiative's large hormone replacement therapy study conducted in the late 1990s was stopped early when it was discovered the combination (estrogen plus progestin) hormone therapy was associated with an increased risk of breast cancer, stroke, and pulmonary embolism. These findings were pivotal for many women, because it highlighted the dangers of traditional oral estrogen/progestin therapy in older women.

In the subsequent WHI Memory Study, researchers found that use of estrogen alone (since the combination proved harmful) did not protect women from normal declines in memory and other cognitive functions when compared with women who took placebo, and in fact women who took estrogen appeared to be at a higher risk for developing dementia than women who took placebo. Note, however, that these findings were seen in women age 65 and older; they may or may not apply to younger women.

A subsequent study has shed some light on the question of whether the impact of estrogen on cognitive function depends on a woman's age. In *Archives of Neurology,* researchers from San Francisco VA Medical Center reported that estrogen therapy may increase or decrease a woman's risk for dementia in later life, depending on when she takes the estrogen.

Dr. Kristine Yaffe, chief of geriatric psychiatry at the VA Medical Center evaluated data from a 40-year period for 5,504 postmenopausal women. She discovered that women who took estrogen therapy in midlife but not in late life had a 26% decreased risk of dementia in old age when compared with women who had never taken estrogen. However, women who took estrogen in old age but not in midlife had a 48% *greater* risk of dementia in old age when compared with women who never took estrogen.

While this is not a definitive study, the findings are certainly food for thought if you ever consider estrogen therapy.

Breast Cancer

The diagnosis of breast cancer is frightening. Even though medicine has made great strides in detecting and treating this disease, learning you have breast cancer and then living with it are life-altering experiences.

Breast cancer forms in the ducts (tubes that transport milk to the nipples) and lobules (glands that produce milk). More than 207,000 women were estimated to have received a diagnosis of breast cancer in 2010, according to the National Cancer Institute. Overall, 1 in 8 women can expect to develop breast cancer at some time during their lives.

Risk Factors for Breast Cancer

Although the exact cause of breast cancer remains unknown, certain risk factors have been identified as making some women more likely to develop the disease than others. Some of these risk factors you cannot change: age (your chance of getting the disease increases with age), race (white women are more likely to get the disease than women of color), family history of breast cancer, the presence of certain genes (e.g., BRCA1 or BRCA2 significantly increase your risk), having dense breast tissue, or having had chest radiation, particularly as a child or adolescent.

Risk factors over which you do have control are consumption of alcohol (the more you drink, the greater your risk), being overweight or obese, lack of exercise, and poor diet. In fact, the World Cancer Research Fund released a new report in February 2011 stating that eating a healthy diet (avoiding refined sugars, processed meats, saturated fat, and fried food, and focusing on fruits, vegetables, whole grains, beans, and energy-dense nuts and seeds), getting regular exercise, and limiting alcohol intake could reduce breast cancer by 38% per year.

Then there are the reproductive and hormonal risk factors, some of which you can control and others you cannot. Your risk of breast cancer is higher if

- You had your first child after age 30.
- You never have children.
- Your first menstrual period began before age 12.
- You go through menopause after age 55.
- You take hormone therapy for 5 or more years for menopause.

The longer estrogens are in your body, the greater your risk of breast cancer. However, as you know, estrogens are also critical for your health, so it is up to you to do all you can to handle the risk factors you can control to minimize your risk of breast cancer.

Preventing Invasive Breast Cancer

Invasive breast cancer is a disease that spreads beyond the milk ducts or lobules into surrounding breast tissue. Two drugs have been shown to help reduce the risk of invasive breast cancer: raloxifene and tamoxifen. Both drugs are known as selective estrogen receptor modulators (SERMs). These drugs block the effects of estrogen on breast tissue and reduce the risk of developing invasive breast cancer because most breast tumors need estrogen to grow.

Tamoxifen has been used for more than 30 years to fight breast cancer and to prevent breast cancer from recurring after initial treatment. Research also shows that the drug may help reduce the risk of both DCIS (ductal carcinoma in situ, a noninvasive breast cancer) and invasive breast cancer in healthy women as well.

Raloxifene (Evista) is perhaps best known as a drug to prevent and treat osteoporosis in women after menopause. Updated results of the 2010 STAR (Study of Tamoxifen and Raloxifene) trial, which involved nearly 20,000 postmenopausal women followed for nearly 7 years during and after they were treated with either tamoxifen or raloxifene, found that 2 years after treatment ended, both tamoxifen and raloxifene reduced the risk of invasive breast cancer by 50% and 38% respectively. Unlike tamoxifen, raloxifene is not used to treat women who already have or have previously had invasive breast cancer. Both of these medications share estrogen's ability to increase the risk for thromboembolic events, so the risks and benefits should be discussed with your health-care provider prior to use.

Treating Breast Cancer

Treatment of breast cancer can take several forms, and many women are involved with more than one treatment option. The options include

- Surgery, including but not limited to lumpectomy and mastectomy.
- Radiation therapy, which often precedes and/or follows surgery.
- Hormone therapy, which stops hormone activity so the cancer will stop growing. It can be used alone or with other treatment options. Examples of hormone therapy for breast cancer include GnRH (gonadotropin-releasing hormone) agonists, which stop production of follicle-stimulating hormone and luteinizing hormone to halt estrogen production by the ovaries in premenopausal women; a class of drugs called aromatase inhibitors: **anastrozole** (Arimidex), exemestane (Aromasin), and **letrozole** (Femara); and an estrogen-blocker called **tamoxifen** (Nolvadex). Because hormone therapy disrupts hormone activity, women taking these medications have a greater risk of osteoporosis, a concern you should discuss with your health-care provider. Interestingly, however, tamoxifen can actually provide some protection against bone loss in women who have already gone through

menopause, although its use has declined since the availability of the somewhat more effective aromatase inhibitor medications.

- Chemotherapy, the use of drugs designed to kill cancer cells but that harm normal cells as well. Chemotherapy can have a significant impact on a woman's menstrual cycle, causing anything from irregular periods to elimination of menstruation altogether. Chemotherapy often also causes nausea, vomiting, hair loss, fatigue, mouth sores, and other symptoms. Some chemotherapy drugs used for breast cancer are in the table below.

- Targeted therapy, which involves drugs, antibodies, or other substances, such as Herceptin, to attack specific cancer cells without harming normal cells. The result is fewer, milder side effects.

One important message concerning breast cancer is that the earlier you identify it, the better your chances of treating—and beating it—successfully. Regular mammograms, breast self-examination, and professional breast exams during your yearly pelvic exams are recommended. Report any abnormalities you find in your breasts to your doctor immediately.

If you have breast cancer, learn all you can about your treatment options and how healthy lifestyle changes can complement them, and work closely with your health-care provider when making treatment decisions, including any medications you take and their side effects and other impacts on your life.

Chemotherapy for Breast Cancer

Both individual chemotherapy drugs and combinations are used to treat breast cancer. These drugs include:

- **cyclophosphamide** (Cytoxan)
- doxorubicin (Adriamycin)
- Fluorouracil (5-FU)
- **Methotrexate**
- ACMF: doxorubicin, followed by a combination of cyclophosphamide, methotrexate, and fluorouracil
- ACT: doxorubicin plus cyclophosphamide, followed by paclitaxel (Taxol) or docetaxel (Taxotere)

- A-T-C: doxorubicin followed by paclitaxel followed by cyclophosphamide

If your breast cancer has spread or come back, the following chemotherapy drugs may be used alone:

- capecitabine (Xeloda)
- **cyclophosphamide**
- docetaxel
- doxorubicin
- epirubicin (Ellence)
- fluorouracil
- gemcitabine
- paclitaxel
- vinorelbine (Navelbine)

Depression

Depression in women and men is not the same, and one of the main reasons for the difference is—you guessed it—hormones. Then there is the fact that more women than men suffer from depression. During their lifetime, 10–25% of women and 5–12% of men will become clinically depressed. Depression affects approximately 19 million Americans, or about 9.5% of the population in any given year.

Scientists have explored the influence of female hormones on brain chemistry, specifically the areas that control emotions and mood. Overall, women are especially vulnerable to depression during times when their hormones are in flux: during puberty; the days before their menstrual period; before, during, and just after pregnancy (postpartum depression); just before and during menopause (perimenopause). If you are thinking, "Hey, that sounds like a big part of my life!" you are right.

Types of Depression in Women

Two conditions often associated with depression are premenstrual dysphoric disorder (PDD), a more severe form of premenstrual syndrome (PMS), and postpartum depression. Symptoms occur during the week just before menstrual bleeding and usually improve within a few days after the period starts. To be given a diagnosis of PDD, the criteria state you should have 5 or more of the following symptoms:

- Feeling hopeless or sad, including suicidal thoughts
- Feelings of anxiety or tension
- Panic attacks
- Lack of interest in daily activities and relationships
- Mood swings accompanied by crying
- Persistent anger or irritability that has an impact on other people
- Fatigue or low energy
- Difficulty concentrating
- Sleep problems
- Food cravings and/or bingeing
- Feeling like you are out of control
- Bloating, breast tenderness, headache, joint or muscle pain

This roller coaster of emotions and physical problems can in itself take a toll on your life, exacerbating depression.

If you suffer from PDD, your hormones are not necessarily "performing" in an unusual way, but you likely have different responses and/or are hypersensitive to your hormone changes. Scientists are still trying to figure out the exact roles of estrogen and other hormones in PDD and PMS.

If you have recently given birth, you are susceptible to postpartum depression, when your hormones and physical changes, along with your new responsibilities, can be overwhelming. Although many new mothers experience a brief case of "baby blues," about 10% suffer from postpartum depression, which requires active treatment with medication, counseling, or both.

Menopause brings its own set of hormonal changes, and for some women the transition into menopause increases their risk for depression. The good news: Depression becomes less common during postmenopause, once the hormones settle down.

Treating Depression

The arsenal available to treat depression is extensive and includes medications in the following drug categories:

- Selective serotonin reuptake inhibitors (SSRIs) are the most commonly prescribed class of drugs for depression. Examples are citalopram

(Celexa), **escitalopram** (Lexapro), **fluoxetine** (Prozac), **paroxetine** (Paxil), and sertraline (Zoloft). The newest addition to this category was approved by the FDA in January 2011, with vilazodone (Vibryd). This drug reportedly is less likely to cause weight gain and loss of sexual desire, which are side effects of many of its rivals in this drug group and others. Some of the side effects associated with SSRIs include dizziness, fatigue, headache, insomnia, sexual problems, and weight changes.

- Serotonin norepinephrine reuptake inhibitors (SNRIs) are the newer type of antidepressant. Drugs in this class include **duloxetine** (Cymbalta), desvenlafaxine (Pristiq), and venlafaxine (Effexor). Common side effects include anxiety, dizziness, fatigue, insomnia, decreased sexual desire, and upset stomach.

- Tricyclic antidepressants are some of the first medications used to treat depression. Among the drugs in this category are **amitriptyline** (Endep), desipramine (Norpramin), doxepin (Sinequan), imipramine (Tofranil), nortriptyline (Aventyl), and trimipramine (Surmontil). Possible side effects include decreased blood pressure and/or blood sugar levels, dizziness, dry mouth, nausea, and stomach upset.

- Monoamine oxidase inhibitors (MAOIs) were among the first drug treatments for depression, but they are not prescribed very often anymore because they carry a high risk of serious side effects. They also react negatively with some foods, including aged cheeses, bananas, chocolate, and wines. Drugs in this category include isocarboxazid (Marplan), phenelzine (Nardil), and selegiline (EMSAM). Side effects include daytime sleepiness, diarrhea, difficulty urinating, dizziness, insomnia, low blood pressure, muscle aches, nervousness, reduced sexual desire, tingling sensation in the skin, and weight gain.

- Other medications occasionally prescribed for depression include bupropion (Wellbutrin), which may be less likely to cause sexual side effects than most other antidepressants. Side effects include anxiety, headache, insomnia, and upset stomach. **Trazodone** (Desyrel) is also prescribed for depression. Its side effects include blurry vision, constipation, dizziness, drowsiness, and dry mouth.

Here are yet a few more concerns about antidepressants. After a review of clinical trials of antidepressants by the FDA in 2004, the agency ordered all antidepressant makers to put a "black box" warning label on their medications about the potential increased risk of suicidal thinking or attempts in young people who took antidepressants. In 2007, that warning was extended to include young adults up through age 24. The warning emphasizes that people of any age who take antidepressants should be monitored closely for worsening depression, suicidal thinking or actions, or any unusual changes in behavior, especially during the first few weeks of taking the medication.

Fibrocystic Breasts

At one time, fibrocystic breasts was called fibrocystic breast disease, but it is not a disease at all. Fibrocystic breasts is a common, benign condition characterized by lumpiness, discomfort, tenderness, and pain in one or both breasts. More than 60% of women experience fibrocystic breasts, and the condition mostly affects women between the ages of 30 and 50. The good news is that fibrocystic breasts tend to resolve significantly after menopause.

The so-called life cycle of fibrocystic breasts is a clue to its main cause: hormones, specifically your normal hormonal fluctuations during your monthly cycle. The primary culprits are estrogen and progesterone, both of which directly impact breast tissue by causing cells to grow and reproduce. But these two hormones do not act alone; growth factor, insulin, prolactin, and thyroid hormone all have some influence on breast tissue. In addition, breast tissue itself produces hormonal substances from fat and glandular cells, and these substances may boost the effects of estrogen and progesterone as well as send signals to other breast cells that may contribute to the symptoms of fibrocystic breasts.

All of this cellular activity in your breasts can contribute to the symptoms of fibrocystic breasts, which can range from mild to severe from month to month, and even vary in different areas of your breasts. **Acetaminophen** and NSAIDs prove helpful for many women, as does wearing a bra at night, warm compresses, and **fish oil supplements.** If your fibrocystic breast symptoms are severe, your health-care provider may recommend oral contraceptives to help reduce the dramatic swings in hormones associated with your menstrual cycle and hopefully suppress your symptoms.

Osteoporosis

For many women, the first clue that they have osteoporosis is when they experience a fall and fracture a bone. That's because osteoporosis, a condition characterized by a decrease in bone density and strength, typically has no symptoms. Out of sight, out of mind, that is, until a broken wrist, arm, or hip, or a compression fracture of the spine occurs.

Bones and Bone Loss

Normal, healthy bone is composed of **calcium,** protein, collagen, and other elements, all of which work together to give bones their strength. Bone density is determined by how much bone is in the skeletal structure, and the higher the bone density, the stronger the bones. Although genetics has a significant role in determining bone density, hormonal, environmental, and lifestyle factors also have a great deal of influence. We will focus on the hormones.

The most important hormone for your bones is estrogen. Bones accumulate density during childhood and adolescence and peak around age 25. After age 35, women (and men) typically lose 0.3–0.5% of their bone density each year. When estrogen levels decline after menopause, however, bone loss in women speeds up considerably, clocking in at about 2–4% loss of density per year for 3–5 years after menopause. This accelerated bone loss in postmenopausal women is a major concern, but also one women can face head-on with diet, exercise, supplements, and medication (if needed).

Medications for Osteoporosis

Our bones are in a constant state of flux, as pockets of old bone tissue are removed and new bone is put in its place. Osteoporosis develops when more bone is removed than can be replaced. The most common medications to prevent and treat osteoporosis are antiresorptive drugs, which reduce the amount of bone tissue that is removed (resorbed) from bones. Commonly used antiresorptive drugs include a class called bisphosphonates, which includes **alendronate** (Fosamax), **ibandronate** (Boniva), **risedronate** (Actonel), and **zoledronic acid** (Reclast). Most of these medications are oral and are available in doses that can be taken daily, weekly, or monthly, depending on the drug. Zoledronic acid is unique in that it is administered only once a year as an infusion. **Denosumab** (Prolia) represents a new class of antiresorptive medications that can be given every 6 months by a simple cutaneous injection in the doctor's office.

Another antiresorptive medication often used to treat osteoporosis is **raloxifene** (Evista), which belongs to a drug class called selective estrogen receptor modulators. Raloxifene is "selective" because it can act like estrogen on bone and thus promote bone density, and also act like an antiestrogen on the breast and uterine lining, protecting these tissues from the cancer-promoting effects of estrogen.

When osteoporosis is advanced, particularly after breaks or fractures have already occurred, use of a medication that increases the production of new bone, such as **teriparatide** (Forteo), is often prescribed for 1–2 years to repair the damage before switching to an antiresorptive medication.

Preventing and treating osteoporosis are critical steps every woman should take. Deciding when medications are needed requires a bone density measurement (generally indicated only for women past menopause) and an individualized assessment of your risk for broken bones in the future. However, if you have already experienced a break of your hip or spine after age 45, you are a definite candidate for treatment. Fifty percent of white women can expect to experience a fracture during their lifetime. Twenty percent of women who have a hip fracture will die in the subsequent year as an indirect result of their fracture, often from an infection or pneumonia. About 20% of postmenopausal women who have a vertebral fracture will suffer a new vertebral fracture in the following year. There are no bones about it: It pays to protect your bone health.

Chapter 6

Prescription Drug Abuse

It's an unfortunate fact that about 4 million women abuse prescription drugs. You may know someone—your best friend, a coworker, your mother, sister, niece, aunt, cousin—who is misusing or abusing a drug that was prescribed for her at one time to address a specific medical need. But now that time has passed, and she is continuing to take the medication. Perhaps that person is even you. Whether you are misusing prescription medication or you know someone who is, *now* is the time to take action. The first step is acknowledging the problem.

In this chapter we take a look at the problem of prescription drug abuse among women, how it can affect your health and the health of your child, and what you can do about it.

First, a Word About Illegal Drug Abuse

Another very serious aspect of drug abuse among women is the use of illegal drugs. Since this book is about prescription medications and not illegal drugs, I do not address this issue except to point out that according to the National Institute on Drug Abuse, about 9 million women in the United States have used illegal drugs within the past year. That's more than twice the number as those who abused prescription drugs. Of these, about 2 million have taken cocaine and 6 million use marijuana. Most women drug abusers take more than one drug, and that may include the use of both illegal and prescription drugs. If you or someone you know is having trouble with illegal drugs, *get help so you (or they) can quit and live a full, productive life.* The National Drug Information Treatment and Referral Line (1-800-662-HELP [4357]) is a good place to start.

Prescription Drug Abuse Among Women

According to the National Institute on Drug Abuse, women are more likely than men to be prescribed an abusable prescription drug, especially benzodiazepines (antianxiety drugs) and opioids (narcotics). Of special concern are women who misuse medications while they are pregnant. Many, if not most, medications have been found to be either definitely or potentially harmful to the fetus, or there is not enough evidence to know if they are dangerous. (This information is provided for each of the drugs discussed in part II of this book.) Abusing prescription medications, however, is especially dangerous for the fetus, and any woman who is pregnant and is misusing medications needs immediate help, both for herself and for her unborn child.

In a May 2010 interview by the NIH's Office of Research on Women's Health, Vivian W. Pinn, MD, director of the office, spoke with Nora Volkow, MD, director of the National Institute on Drug Abuse. Dr. Volkow pointed out that some people believe that abuse of prescription drugs is less dangerous than abuse of illicit drugs because they have been prescribed by doctors. Abuse of drugs such as Vicodin or OxyContin, as well as stimulants, however, can lead to addiction.

Using imaging studies, Dr. Volkow has shown that repeated drug use disrupts the circuits of the brain that are involved with learning and with the ability to feel pleasure, as well as in areas that are responsible for decision making, judgment, and controlling your emotions and desires. She stressed that "when you take psychotherapeutics outside the surveillance of a physician, these medications can be as dangerous as illicit substances." And prescription drug use can get out of control insidiously and quickly.

The Drugs of Abuse

The National Institute on Drug Abuse has identified three classes of prescription drugs that are most often abused: opioids, depressants, and stimulants. Topping the list are opioids, but benzodiazepines (a type of depressant) come in a close second.

Opioids

Opioids are potent narcotic painkillers that are often prescribed to treat pain after surgery or a medical or dental procedure. Common drugs in this category include propoxyphene (Darvon), meperidine (Demerol), hydromorphone (Dilaudid), diphenoxylate (Lomotil), **oxycodone** (OxyContin), and **hydrocodone/acetaminophen** (Vicodin). Codeine is often prescribed for mild to moderate pain, while codeine and diphenoxylate are frequently prescribed to treat diarrhea and coughs. When opioids are prescribed by a physician and used as directed, they are generally safe and do not lead to addictive behavior. However, opioids can quickly trigger addiction if you misuse them.

One of the dangers of opioids is the fact that they act directly on the respiratory center in the brain stem, which means they can slow your breathing. An overdose of opioids can cause your respiratory centers to shut down completely, with the result being death. They can also have a negative impact on your cardiovascular system and nervous system, causing decreased consciousness, euphoria, and confusion.

Another danger is combining opioids with other substances that depress the central nervous system, such as alcohol, antihistamines, barbiturates, benzodiazepines, or general anesthetics. These combinations can be life-threatening. If you are misusing prescription opioids, you need to talk to your health-care provider about how to safely taper off these drugs to avoid withdrawal symptoms—and worse.

Depressants

Depressants, which are sometimes referred to as sedatives and tranquilizers, act directly on your central nervous system and slow down normal brain function. Drugs in this category include barbiturates such as pentobarbital (Nembutal), which is used to treat anxiety, tension, and sleep problems;

and benzodiazepines, such as **alprazolam** (Xanax), chlordiazepoxide (Librium), and **diazepam** (Valium), which are prescribed to treat anxiety, acute stress reactions, and panic attacks. Some of the more sedating benzodiazepines, such as triazolam (Halcion) and estazolam (ProSom) are often prescribed for sleep problems. Generally, benzodiazepines are not prescribed for long-term use, but unfortunately some women take them for far too long.

All of these and other central nervous system depressants are highly addictive. Use of these depressants along with other medications or substances that cause central nervous system depression, such as prescription pain medications, some OTC cold and allergy medications, and alcohol, can be especially dangerous. Any of these combinations can slow both your breathing and heart rate and even cause your death. If you have been taking any of these drugs for a prolonged time, you should talk to your health-care provider about how you can *safely* stop them (but *never* stop cold turkey).

Stimulants

Stimulants are occasionally abused because women use them for weight loss. There are much safer ways to lose weight! Drugs such as dextroamphetamine (Adderall, Dexedrine) and methylphenidate (Concerta, Ritalin) are chemically similar to brain neurotransmitters called monoamines. These stimulants enhance the effects of these neurotransmitters and also cause a rise in blood pressure and heart rate, constrict blood vessels, increase blood glucose, and open up airways in your lungs. They also cause a sense of euphoria.

Stimulants are not prescribed as much for adults as they are for children (for attention-deficit/hyperactivity disorder), but there is still the potential for misuse. Withdrawal symptoms associated with stopping stimulant use include depression, fatigue, and problems with sleep. Repeated use of some stimulants over a short period of time may cause you to feel hostility or paranoia, while high doses may cause dangerously high body temperature, irregular heartbeat, fatal seizures, and cardiovascular failure.

"Neither a Borrower, nor a Lender Be"

When considering prescription drugs, Shakespeare's admonition is good advice, as a problem related and contributing to drug abuse is women sharing or borrowing prescription drugs. In a survey of nearly 7,500 women ages 18–44 that was published in the *Journal of Women's Health,* it was reported that

36.5% of women in this age group said they had ever borrowed or shared prescription medications. Topping the list of drugs were allergy medications (43.8%) and painkillers (42.6%).

This is a dangerous practice because of possible unanticipated side effects or drug-drug interactions, complications from using the drugs incorrectly, and risk of addiction. Another problem is women who become pregnant, who are pregnant, or who are breast-feeding and using these drugs without their doctor's knowledge. According to Susan G. Kornstein, MD, executive director of the Virginia Commonwealth University Institute for Women's Health, "It is clear that patients need to be counseled about the potential risks of sharing and borrowing medications, especially if they are women of reproductive age."

Men and Women Are Different

Okay, I have stated the obvious, but when it comes to prescription drugs, men and women misuse or abuse them for different reasons. A 2010 Harvard study looked at the role that gender plays in the risk for abuse of prescription pain medications. The study participants included 662 men and women who had noncancer-related chronic pain and who had been prescribed opioid pain medication.

The researchers surveyed each participant with standard pain assessment questionnaires that examined rates and characteristics of problem opioid use, risk factors for potential misuse, and predictive associations between risk factors and eventual misuse of drugs.

The lead researcher, Robert N. Jamison, PhD, a clinical psychologist at Harvard's Brigham and Women's Hospital, reported that while men and women were similar in their frequency of prescription drug abuse, the reasons why they abused them were different. Women were motivated more by emotional and psychological issues while men were more likely to abuse the drugs because of social and behavioral problems. For example, women were more likely to abuse drugs because of problems with their children or their relationships, while men were more likely to abuse because of legal difficulties or because they associated with others who are prone to use addictive substances, such as attending Alcoholics Anonymous meetings.

Jamison and his colleagues also found that women who abuse pain medications are more likely to have been physically or sexually abused, or to have a history of psychological or psychiatric problems. These findings led the study's authors to recommend that women who are being treated with opioids for chronic noncancer pain and who have evidence of significant stress or psychological disorders be treated for their mood and emotional condition and be counseled on the dangers of relying on opioids to deal with their stress.

If you have a history of psychological, sexual, or physical abuse and are misusing prescription drugs, it is critical that you inform a medical professional about your abusive past so you can get proper psychological help, and then work on stopping the medication abuse.

It's Time to Quit

If you are battling a prescription drug problem, you don't need to fight it alone. Chances are you are already trying to deal with mood swings and emotional distress, and you may be facing financial worries and anxiety about getting your drugs as well. Prescription drug misuse often has a negative impact on personal relationships with partners, children, and friends, even causing them to fall apart, while a woman's health can suffer irreparable damage.

The first step to stopping prescription drug abuse is acknowledging you have a problem, and then seeking help from someone you trust: a physician, spiritual leader, friend, relative, or mental-health professional. There are treatment programs and options for every financial situation and personal need. One place to start is with the National Drug Information Treatment and Referral Line (1-800-662-HELP [4357]). But nothing will happen unless you take the initiative.

Part Two

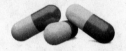

Drug and Supplement Profiles

Acetaminophen

Brand Names
> Panadol, Tylenol

Available as Generic?
> Yes

Principal Uses
> Fever; aches and pains related to a variety of conditions, including but not limited to arthritis, headache, colds, and flu

About the Drug
> Acetaminophen is an analgesic (pain reliever) and antipyretic (fever reducer). Acetaminophen relieves pain by raising your pain threshold; that is, it allows your body to withstand a greater level of pain before you feel it. Although acetaminophen can relieve pain, it has no effect on inflammation, redness, or swelling, as do NSAIDs such as ibuprofen. Acetaminophen reduces fever by acting on the heat-controlling center of the brain, instructing it to lower your body's temperature when your temperature rises.

How to Use This Drug
> Acetaminophen is available over the counter in the form of chewable tablets, coated caplets, gelcaps, geltabs, liquid, and suppositories. The typical oral dose for adults is 325–650 mg every 4–6 hours, with a maximum daily dose of 4 grams. The adult dose for the suppository is 650 mg every 4–6 hours.

> When using the liquid form, shake the bottle well before each dose, and measure the liquid with the device provided with the medication. Chew the chewable tablets thoroughly before you swallow them. If you take rapidly dissolving tablets, you can chew them or allow them to dissolve and then swallow with or without water. The sustained-release tablets must be taken whole; do not chew, crush, or break them.

> You should not take acetaminophen for longer than 3 days if you are treating a fever or for more than 10 days if treating pain, unless your doctor has instructed you otherwise.

Side Effects
- When used as directed, acetaminophen rarely causes side effects.
- Rare but very serious side effects: abdominal pain, dark urine, easy bruising or bleeding, extreme tiredness, new signs of infection (e.g., fever, persistent sore throat), persistent nausea and/or vomiting, and yellowing of the skin or eyes.

Possible Drug, Supplement, and/or Food Interactions

- Chronic use of alcohol or other drugs that can damage the liver, while taking acetaminophen, can result in serious liver damage and/or an increased risk of stomach bleeding.
- Carbamazepine, isoniazid, and rifampin may reduce the levels of acetaminophen and thus decrease its action.
- Cholestyramine reduces the effects of acetaminophen by decreasing your body's ability to absorb it. Therefore, acetaminophen should be taken 3–4 hours after or 1 hour before taking cholestyramine.
- Taking more than 2275 mg per day of acetaminophen may increase the ability of warfarin to thin your blood.

Tell Your Doctor

- About any allergies you have and all OTC and prescription medications you are taking, as well as supplements.
- If you regularly use alcohol and/or have liver disease, because acetaminophen may cause liver damage.
- If you have diabetes, phenylketonuria, or any condition that requires you to limit or avoid sugar or aspartame. Some acetaminophen products contain these substances.
- Use of acetaminophen may interfere with the results of various lab tests. Be sure to tell your health-care provider and lab personnel you are taking acetaminophen.

Of Special Interest to Women

- Although acetaminophen is typically used in all stages of pregnancy and is considered safe for short-term treatment of fever and minor pain, you should still consult your doctor before taking acetaminophen if you are pregnant.
- Acetaminophen passes into breast milk. Although use of acetaminophen while nursing appears to be safe, consult your doctor before you breast-feed.

Symptoms of Overdose

Dark urine, extreme tiredness, increased sweating, nausea, severe abdominal pain, vomiting, and yellowing of the eyes or skin.

Acyclovir

Brand Name
Zovirax

Available as Generic?

Yes

Principal Uses

Cold sores (herpes simplex 1), genital herpes (herpes simplex 2), shingles (varicella-zoster), mononucleosis (Epstein-Barr)

About the Drug

Acyclovir is one of a group of antiviral drugs that are effective against the herpes viruses, including herpes simplex 1 and 2 (HSV-1, HSV-2), varicella-zoster, and Epstein-Barr. Genital HSV-2 infection is twice as common in women than in men. (Two other antiviral drugs used to treat herpes viruses are famciclovir [Famvir] and valacyclovir [Valtrex].) Acyclovir inhibits the replication of DNA that the virus needs to reproduce and survive. Cells that are infected with the virus absorb more acyclovir than unaffected cells and then convert more of the drug to an active form, which in turn prolongs its antiviral activity.

How to Use the Drug

Acyclovir is available in capsules, tablets, powder for injection, suspension, and ointment. You can take the oral forms with or without food. The typical oral adult dose is 200–800 mg every 4 hours; the usual adult intravenous dose is 5–10 mg/kg every 8 hours for 7 days. When taking the oral dose, drink lots of fluids unless your doctor tells you otherwise. If using the liquid form, shake the bottle well before each dose and measure the dose using the special measuring spoon that comes with the prescription.

The oral doses reduce the pain and the number of lesions in an initial outbreak of genital herpes, and can decrease the frequency and severity of recurrent bouts. When treating shingles, acyclovir can reduce pain and healing time while also limiting the spread of the virus and development of new lesions. Intravenous acyclovir is used to treat herpes simplex and chicken pox in people who are immunocompromised. Topical acyclovir is used to treat initial genital herpes to reduce pain and healing time, and to limit spread of the infection.

Side Effects

- Most common side effects: diarrhea, headache, nausea, and vomiting.
- Less common side effects: agitation, anemia, confusion, muscle pain, and rash. There have also been reports of seizures and hepatitis.
- Contact your doctor immediately if you experience a change in the amount of urine, unusual back and/or side pain, mental changes (e.g., confusion, hallucinations), shaky and/or unsteady movement,

trouble speaking, abnormal heartbeat, easy bruising and/or bleeding, new fever, severe abdominal pain, jaundice, loss of consciousness, or seizures.

Possible Drug, Supplement, and/or Food Interactions

- Acyclovir may reduce levels of phenytoin (Dilantin) or valproic acid (Depakote).
- Acyclovir may increase serum levels of theophylline (Theo-Dur).
- Probenecid (Benemid) may increase acyclovir serum levels.
- The herb astragalus can increase the immune effects of acyclovir.

Tell Your Doctor

- About all prescription and OTC medications you are taking, as well as supplements.
- If you have a history of kidney problems or any condition related to a compromised immune system (e.g., kidney transplant, bone marrow transplant, HIV).
- If you are allergic to acyclivor or valacyclovir, or if you have any other allergies.

Of Special Interest to Women

- No adequate studies of the impact of acyclovir in pregnant women have been done. However, in a patient registry of pregnant women who used acyclovir during the first trimester, the birth defect rate was similar to that seen in the general population.
- Acyclovir is excreted in breast milk, and infants can receive a significant amount of this drug via breast-feeding. Although acyclovir is not believed to harm nursing infants, talk to your doctor before you begin breast-feeding.
- This drug does not protect against the spread of genital herpes. Therefore, to reduce your chance of giving herpes to your partner, do not have sexual contact during an outbreak of the disease or while you are experiencing symptoms. Because you can also spread the virus when you do not have symptoms, you should use an effective barrier (e.g., condoms) during sexual activity.

Symptoms of Overdose

Agitation, changes in the amount of urine, fatigue, loss of consciousness, and seizures.

Alendronate

Brand Names
Fosamax, Fosamax Plus D

Available as Generic?
Yes

Principal Uses
Prevention and treatment of osteoporosis; also Paget's disease

About the Drug
Alendronate is prescribed to prevent and treat osteoporosis (bone loss) in women who have undergone menopause. It is also prescribed for women who are taking corticosteroids (medications that may cause osteoporosis), and to treat Paget's disease of the bone, a condition in which bones are soft and may be deformed, painful, or easily fractured.

Alendronate belongs to the drug class bisphosphonates, medications that decrease the activity of cells called osteoclasts, which break down bone, and help increase bone density. Alendronate also helps reduce the risk of fractures. (See, however, the warning about alendronate under "Of Special Interest to Women" below.) Some other bisphosphonates are etidronate (Didronel), ibandronate (Boniva), risedronate (Actonel), and zoledronic acid (Reclast, Zometa).

How to Use This Drug
Alendronate is available in tablets and liquid solution. The recommended dose for treating osteoporosis is 5–10 mg daily or 35–70 mg weekly. For Paget's disease, the typical dose is 40 mg once daily for 6 months. Take all your doses on an empty stomach immediately after rising in the morning. Never take alendronate at bedtime, before you get out of bed, or any other part of the day.

The liquid is usually taken once a week in the morning. Swallow at least 2 ounces of plain water after taking the liquid dose. The 5 mg and 10 mg tablets are usually taken once daily, and the 35 mg and 70 mg tablets are usually taken once a week. Take the tablets with 6–8 ounces of plain water; do not use juice, sparkling water, tea, or any other liquid. Do not chew, split, suck, or crush the tablets; they must be swallowed whole.

Sit or stand upright for at least 30 minutes after taking your dose. Do not eat, drink, or take any other medications or supplements for at least 30 minutes. It is important to follow the dosing directions exactly, or you may experience side effects.

Side Effects
- Most common side effect: stomach pain.
- Less common side effects: black stools, bloating, constipation, diarrhea, gas, joint or muscle pain, nausea, taste changes, and vomiting.
- Alendronate may irritate the esophagus and cause bleeding and ulcers if you do not take the drug exactly as directed.
- Rarely, alendronate causes jaw problems associated with delayed healing and infection after tooth extraction.
- If you experience any of the following symptoms, contact your doctor immediately before you take any more alendronate: new or worsening heartburn, difficult or painful swallowing, chest pain, bloody or coffee-ground-like vomit, black or blood stools, fever, blisters, peeling skin, hives, hoarseness, loosening of the teeth, numbness or heavy jaw, eye pain, painful or swollen gums, or swelling of eyes, face, lips, tongue, or throat.

Possible Drug, Supplement, and/or Food Interactions
- All food and other medications or supplements may interfere with the absorption of alendronate, so they should be consumed no sooner than 30 minutes after you take alendronate.
- Calcium supplements and antacids reduce the absorption of alendronate. Therefore, take alendronate at least 30 minutes before calcium and antacids.
- Aspirin or other NSAIDs along with alendronate may increase the risk of stomach and intestinal side effects.
- Intravenous ranitidine (Zantac) increases the blood levels of alendronate, although the impact of this interaction is not known.

Tell Your Doctor
- If you have any allergies and all OTC and prescription medications you are taking, as well as supplements.
- If you are not able to remain upright for at least 30 minutes after taking this medication.
- If you have any abnormalities of the esophagus that can delay esophageal emptying, such as stricture or poor motility (achalasia). If you do, you should not take this medication.
- If you are taking any of the following prescription or OTC medications, as your doctor may need to change the doses of your medications or watch you for side effects: aspirin and other NSAIDs, cancer chemotherapy, oral steroids (e.g., dexamethasone), methylprednisolone, and prednisone.

- If you are undergoing radiation therapy, have or have a history of anemia, low vitamin D levels, kidney disease, heartburn, ulcers or other stomach problems, cancer, difficulty swallowing, blood-clotting problems, or any dental disease.

- Immediately if you experience severe bone, muscle, or joint pain while taking alendronate. This type of pain can occur within days, months, or even years after you first take alendronate, so it is important to report such pain so your doctor can determine its cause. He or she may tell you to stop taking alendronate.

- Tell your dentist that you plan to take the medication and have your teeth examined. If you need any dental treatment, it should be completed before starting alendronate, as the drug may cause serious problems with your jaw, especially if you have dental surgery or treatments.

Of Special Interest to Women

- The FDA has added a special warning to the labels for alendronate and other bisphosphonates regarding uncommon fractures that may be associated with use of these drugs. These include subtrochanteric femur fractures, which occur in the bone just below the hip joint; and diaphyseal femur fractures, which occur in the long part of the thigh bone. These fractures make up less than 1% of all femur and hip fractures. Although it is not clear whether bisphosphonates cause these unusual fractures, they have been predominantly found in patients who take bisphosphonates.

- It can take 3 months or longer after starting treatment before bone density begins to increase. Alendronate works only if you take it regularly.

- Talk to your doctor if you are pregnant, plan to get pregnant, or are breast-feeding. Alendronate may remain in the body for years after you stop treatment. The effect of alendronate on the fetus is not known, nor is it known whether this drug passes into breast milk.

Symptoms of Overdose

Bloody or black stools, difficulty swallowing, heartburn, nausea, painful swallowing, and stomach pain.

Allopurinol

Brand Names
  Aloprim, Zyloprim
Available as Generic?
  Yes
Principal Uses
  Gout, kidney stones, gouty joint disease, gouty kidney disease
About the Drug
  Allopurinol is prescribed to treat gout, which is caused by high levels of uric acid (hyperuricemia) that accumulate in the joints, most often the big toe, as well as the anklebones and knees. Uric acid forms as a by-product of the metabolism of proteins called purines. Hyperuricemia develops when the body makes more uric acid than it can eliminate. High uric acid levels can also cause kidney stones and kidney disease.

  Allopurinol is a xanthine oxidase inhibitor. The drug prevents the production of uric acid by blocking the activity of the enzyme that changes purines into uric acid. Levels of uric acid usually begin to decline 2–3 days after treatment starts, but it does not become fully effective until it is taken for 2–3 months. Allopurinol will help prevent gout attacks but will not help an attack once it has started.

How to Use This Drug
  Allopurinol is available as tablets, which are usually taken once or twice daily, preferably after a meal. Typically, doctors start patients at a low dose and gradually increase it as necessary. The dose range is 100–800 mg daily. It may take several months before you feel the full benefits of allopurinol. During the first few months, the drug may increase the number of gout attacks that you experience, and your doctor may prescribe another medication during this time until allopurinol begins to prevent the attacks.

  Drink at least 8 glasses of water or other fluids daily while taking allopurinol unless your doctor instructs you otherwise. The fluids help prevent the formation of kidney stones.

Side Effects
  - Common side effects: diarrhea, drowsiness, itching, rash, and upset stomach.
  - Less common side effects, which you should report to your doctor: blood in the urine, painful urination, chills, fever, irritated eyes,

itching, loss of appetite, rash, swelling of the lips or mouth, and unexpected weight loss.

Possible Drug, Supplement, and/or Food Interactions

- Alcohol may reduce the effectiveness of allopurinol.
- Allopurinol increases blood levels of oral mercaptopurine and azathioprine.
- Allopurinol with penicillins increases the risk of rash.

Tell Your Doctor

- If you have any allergies and all OTC and prescription medications you are taking, as well as supplements.
- If you are taking any of the following medications: amoxicillin, ampicillin, anticoagulants, cancer chemotherapy, chlorpropamide, diuretics, drugs that suppress the immune system such as azathioprine and cyclosporine, other drugs for gout such as probenecid, and tolbutamide. Use of any of these medications with allopurinol may require your doctor to adjust the doses of your drugs.
- If you have ever had liver disease, kidney disease, diabetes, hypertension, or heart failure, or if you have a history of fasting.

Of Special Interest to Women

- The effects of allopurinol on pregnant women and their infant are not known. Consult your health-care provider about the benefits and risks of using allopurinol while pregnant.
- Allopurinol is excreted in breast milk; therefore, discuss the benefits and risks of breast-feeding with your physician.

Symptoms of Overdose

The common side effects, although they will be more severe.

Alosetron

Brand Name

Lotronex

Available as Generic?

No

Principal Use

Irritable bowel syndrome

About the Drug

Alosetron is approved for treating women who have irritable bowel syndrome (IBS) that has diarrhea (rather than constipation) as its main symptom and who have not responded to conventional therapy for IBS. This drug is classified as a 5-HT3 serotonin receptor blocker. (Other drugs in this class are dolasetron, granisetron, and ondansetron.) Serotonin and its receptors in the intestinal tract appear to control how pain is felt, the contraction of muscles in the intestinal tract, and the release of fluid into the intestines. In people who have IBS, it is believed that food, medications, stress, and hormonal changes may trigger an excessive amount of serotonin or an abnormal response to it. Alosetron blocks 5-HT3 receptors and thus reduces the activity of serotonin.

Alosetron was withdrawn from the market in November 2000 after reports of life-threatening gastrointestinal side effects. It was reinstated by the FDA in June 2002, but it is now allowed only for women who have severe, diarrhea-dominant IBS and have not responded to conventional treatment. Studies show that alosetron can provide adequate relief from abdominal pain and discomfort in 40% of patients.

How to Use This Drug

This drug is dispensed for specially selected patients only. Alosetron is available in tablets, and the usual dose is 1 mg twice daily with or without food. Do not begin to take alosetron if you are constipated; consult your physician before beginning treatment.

Side Effects

- Most common side effect: constipation, which can develop in up to one-third of patients.
- Less common side effects: abdominal distension, hemorrhoids, and nausea.
- Rarely, alosetron causes ischemic colitis, a life-threatening condition characterized by severe intestinal inflammation caused by poor blood circulation. Seek immediate medical attention if you experience sudden worsening of abdominal pain and rectal bleeding.
- Tell your doctor immediately if you experience bloating or depression while using alosetron.
- Stop using alosetron immediately if you experience unexplained fever, bloody stools, unusually fast pulse, sudden worsening of abdominal and/or bowel pain, or severe constipation.

Possible Drug, Supplement, and/or Food Interactions

- Alosetron may affect several enzymes in the liver that are involved in the elimination of other drugs, which means it may increase or decrease the blood levels of those other drugs. However, only a few drugs have been tested, and so it is not certain which drugs are involved.

Some that may be affected by alosetron are isoniazid, procainamide, MAOIs, and hydralazine.

- Serious interactions may occur if you use alosetron with apomorphine or fluvoxamine.
- Some medications can affect the elimination of alosetron from the body, which can impact how alosetron works. These drugs include cimetidine, quinolone, and antibiotics.

Tell Your Doctor

- If you have any allergies and about all prescription and OTC drugs you are taking, as well as supplements.
- If you have any of the following medical conditions, because you should not take alosetron if you do: certain intestinal disorders (e.g., ileus, ischemic colitis, impaired intestinal circulation, constipation or its complications, intestinal obstruction, megacolon, perforation, stricture/adhesions), Crohn's disease, ulcerative colitis, diverticulitis, severe liver disease, blood disorders.
- Before using any medication that could slow down the gut and cause constipation, such as sleep aids, allergy medications, and cough and cold products.

Of Special Interest to Women

- No studies of alosetron have been done in pregnant women. You and your health-care provider should discuss the benefits and risks of using alosetron during pregnancy.
- It is not known whether alosetron is excreted in breast milk. You and your health-care provider should discuss the benefits and risks of using alosetron if you are breast-feeding.
- Alosetron is available only for women who have severe diarrhea-predominant IBS and who are prescribed the medication after careful consideration by their health-care provider. Therefore, do not buy alosetron over the Internet. The alosetron your doctor can prescribe for you will come with a risk management program that will fully inform you of the risks and possible benefits of the drug.

Symptoms of Overdose

Difficulty breathing, tremors, seizures, and loss of coordination.

Alprazolam

Brand Name

Xanax

Available as Generic?

Yes

Principal Uses

Anxiety disorders and panic attacks; also depression

About the Drug

Alprazolam is a benzodiazepine, which is one of the top two most frequently abused classes of prescription drugs in the United States (opioids are the other class), according to the Drug Abuse Warning Network. Benzodiazepines are also among the prescription drugs most abused by women. Some other benzodiazepines are clonazepam (Klonopin), diazepam (Valium), flurazepam (Dalmane), lorazepam (Ativan), and temazepan (Restoril).

Alprazolam affects the brain and central nervous system by boosting the influence of the brain chemical GABA (gamma-aminobutyric acid), which inhibits abnormal excitement in the brain. Experts believe that excessive brain activity may lead to anxiety.

How to Use This Drug

Alprazolam is available as tablets and a concentration liquid. It is typically taken 2–4 times daily. If you take the liquid, use the dropper that comes with your prescription. You can add the drug to a small amount of liquid or soft food such as pudding or applesauce; the concentrated liquid will blend completely with food. Drink or eat the entire mixture immediately after preparing it.

Alprazolam can be habit-forming, so never take more than your doctor has prescribed or for longer periods of time. If you want to stop taking alprazolam, talk to your doctor about how to gradually reduce your dose. Suddenly stopping alprazolam can cause symptoms of withdrawal, such as anxiousness, irritability, seizures, and sleeplessness.

Side Effects

- Common side effects: changes in appetite, changes in sexual desire, constipation, dizziness, drowsiness, dry mouth, increased saliva production, light-headedness, tiredness, trouble concentrating, unsteadiness, weight changes.
- Severe side effects, which should be reported to your physician: allergic reactions (e.g., breathing difficulty; hives; itching; rash; swelling of the mouth, face, lips, tongue), confusion, decreased urination, fainting, hallucinations, loss of coordination, memory problems, menstrual changes, mental or mood changes, muscle twitching, seizures, severe dizziness, skin changes (e.g., peeling, blistering, swollen), suicidal thoughts or actions, trouble speaking, yellowing of the skin or eyes.

Possible Drug, Supplement, and/or Food Interactions

- Avoid grapefruit and grapefruit juice when taking alprazolam.
- If you are taking any of the following medications with alprazolam, your doctor may need to change your doses or monitor you for side effects: amiodarone, antidepressants, antifungals, antihistamines, cimetidine, clarithromycin, cyclosporine, diltiazem, ergotamine, erythromycin, isoniazid, medications for mental illness and seizures, nicardipine, nifedipine, SSRIs, sedatives, sleeping pills, and tranquilizers.
- CYP3A inhibitors can increase the concentration and half-life of alprazolam and also decrease its elimination from the body, all of which can cause more significant side effects and other adverse reactions to alprazolam. CYP3A inhibitors include fluoxetine, propoxyphene, and oral contraceptives.
- Do not use Saint-John's-wort when taking alprazolam, as the combination may cause undesirable or dangerous side effects.

Tell Your Doctor

- If you have any allergies, especially to the following drugs: chlordiazepoxide, clonazepam, clorazepate, diazepam, estazolam, flurazepam, halazepam, lorazepam, oxazepam, prazepam, quazepam, temazepam, or triazolam. Also tell him or her all OTC and prescription medications you are taking, as well as supplements.
- If you are taking itraconzazole or ketoconazole. Your doctor will likely not prescribe alprazolam for you.
- If you have or ever had glaucoma; depression; or lung, kidney, or liver disease.
- If you plan to have surgery, including dental surgery, tell your doctor or dentist that you are taking alprazolam.
- If you are taking alprazolam and become pregnant, tell your doctor immediately.

Of Special Interest to Women

- Alprazolam is sometimes prescribed to treat anxiety associated with premenstrual syndrome, as physical symptoms such as weight gain and cramping and emotional symptoms such as feeling out of control can cause anxiety. However, because alprazolam can become addictive if used continuously, relieving PMS symptoms with the use of anti-anxiety medication such as alprazolam should be discussed with your doctor.
- Although no birth defects have been attributed to the use of alprazolam during human pregnancy, the use of other benzodiazepines

are believed to be responsible for fetal abnormalities after first-trimester exposure. In animal studies, alprazolam has been associated with defects when given at the highest dose.

- Alprazolam is excreted in breast milk and has the potential to affect a nursing infant's neurodevelopment. Therefore, do not use alprazolam if you are breast-feeding.

Symptoms of Overdose

Coma, confusion, drowsiness, and problems with coordination.

Amitriptyline

Brand Name

Endep

Available as Generic?

Yes

Principal Uses

Depression; also for fibromyalgia, irritable bowel syndrome, migraine, multiple sclerosis, chronic fatigue syndrome, insomnia, post-traumatic stress disorder, chronic pain, and shingles

About the Drug

Amitriptyline is a tricyclic antidepressant. Other drugs in this class are desipramine (Norpramin), imipramine (Tofranil), nortriptyline (Pamelor), and protriptyline (Vivactil). Amitriptyline elevates mood by raising the level of chemicals in the brain called neurotransmitters, which are involved with mood.

How to Use This Drug

Amitriptyline is available in tablets and can be taken with or without food. The recommended dose is 40–150 mg daily in divided doses. Your doctor will likely start you on a low dose and gradually increase it to the lowest one that is effective.

It may take a few weeks or longer before you experience the full benefits of amitriptyline. Do not suddenly stop taking amitriptyline, as you may experience withdrawal symptoms, including dizziness, headache, nausea, and restlessness. Some people experience these symptoms even if they miss a few doses.

Side Effects

- Common side effects: blurry vision, constipation, dry mouth, fast heart rate, low blood pressure, urinary retention, and weight loss or gain.

- Rare but serious side effects that you should report to your health-care provider immediately: crushing chest pain; fainting or dizziness; hallucinations; hepatitis; hives; rapid heartbeat; rash; seizures; spasms of the jaw, neck, or back; speech difficulties; swelling of the face and tongue; unusual bleeding or bruising; weakness or numbness of the arms or legs; and yellowing of the skin or eyes.
- Use amitriptyline with caution if you have seizures because it can increase your risk of additional seizures.
- Amitriptyline may raise pressure in your eyes if you have glaucoma.
- A small number of young individuals (up to 24 years of age) who have taken antidepressants such as amitriptyline have become suicidal. If you are a young woman taking amitriptyline, contact your health-care professional immediately if you experience any suicidal thoughts.
- Rarely, amitriptyline can cause serotonin syndrome, a serious condition characterized by hallucinations; loss of coordination; severe nausea, vomiting, and diarrhea; twitching muscles; unexplained fever; and unusual restlessness. Seek immediate medical attention if these symptoms occur.
- In rare cases, amitriptyline can cause neuroleptic malignant syndrome, a serious condition characterized by muscle stiffness, severe confusion, sweating, and unexplained fever. Seek immediate medical attention if these symptoms occur.
- Amitriptyline may cause QT prolongation, a condition that affects heart rhythm. QT prolongation infrequently results in serious and even fatal symptoms such as severe dizziness and irregular heartbeat that require immediate medical attention.
- If you have diabetes, amitriptyline may make it more difficult for you to control your blood sugar levels. Be sure to monitor your blood sugar levels regularly.

Possible Drug, Supplement, and/or Food Interactions

- Amitriptyline should not be used with MAOIs. At least a 2-week gap should be maintained between use of amitripytline and MAOIs because of the risk of high fever, convulsions, and death.
- Epinephrine with amitriptyline can result in severe high blood pressure.
- Alcohol with amitriptyline blocks the drug's antidepressant effects but also increases its sedative impact.
- Cimetidine can increase the blood levels of amitriptyline and its side effects.

Tell Your Doctor
- About any allergies, including allergies to other antidepressants, and about all prescription and OTC medications and supplements you are taking.
- If you have stopped taking fluoxetine (Prozac) in the past 5 weeks. Your doctor may need to alter the doses of your medications or watch you for side effects.
- If you have recently had a heart attack, if you drink a large amount of alcohol, or if you have glaucoma, difficulty urinating, seizures, an overactive thyroid (hyperthyroidism), diabetes, schizophrenia, heart problems (including QT prolongation, heart failure, slow heartbeat), liver disease, or kidney disease.
- If you have a personal or family history of mental/mood conditions (e.g., bipolar disorder, psychosis) or suicidal thoughts or behaviors.
- If you plan to have surgery, including dental surgery, tell your doctor or dentist that you are taking amitriptyline.
- If you become pregnant while taking amitriptyline.

Of Special Interest to Women
- It is not known whether amitriptyline is harmful to a fetus. Consult your physician about the benefits and risks of using amitriptyline during pregnancy.
- Amitriptyline is secreted in human milk and may have a harmful effect on nursing infants.

Symptoms of Overdose
Agitation, cold body temperature, coma, confusion, drowsiness, fever, hallucinations, irregular heartbeat, rigid muscles, seizures, and vomiting.

Amlodipine

Brand Name
Norvasc
Available as Generic?
Yes
Principal Uses
Angina, high blood pressure
About the Drug
Amlodipine is a calcium channel blocker, which blocks the movement of calcium into the muscle cells that line the coronary arteries and other

arteries in the body. Other calcium channel blockers include diltiazem (Cardizem), felodipine (Plendil), nicardipine (Cardene), and verapamil (Calan).

Calcium is an important component in muscle contraction; therefore, blocking calcium allows the artery muscles to relax, which facilitates better blood flow. This action prevents chest pain that results when coronary arteries spasm, and it relaxes the muscles lining the arteries throughout the body, which reduces blood pressure. Amlodipine is frequently used along with other medications to treat high blood pressure.

How to Use This Drug

Amlodipine is available as tablets that can be taken with or without food, or as directed. Your physician will base your dose on your health condition and how you respond to treatment. For angina, amlodipine must be taken regularly to be effective. Do not use amlodipine to treat angina only when it occurs.

Side Effects

- Common side effects: edema (swelling) of the lower extremities and headache.
- Less common side effects: dizziness, fatigue, flushing, nausea, and palpitations.
- Unlikely but serious side effects that should be reported to your physician immediately: fainting, fast or irregular heartbeat, and vision changes.
- In people who have severe coronary artery disease, amlodipine may increase the frequency and severity of angina or cause a heart attack.

Possible Drug, Supplement, and/or Food Interactions

- Amlodipine with cough and cold products, diet aids, and NSAIDs (e.g., ibuprofen) may increase your blood pressure or heart rate.
- Consumption of grapefruit or grapefruit juice may increase the concentration of amlodipine.
- Itraconazole with amlodipine may increase the risk of ventricular dysfunction, congestive heart failure, and peripheral and pulmonary edema.
- Tizanidine with amlodipine may cause an excessive drop in blood pressure.

Tell Your Doctor

- If you have any allergies, and all OTC and prescription medications you are taking (especially conivaptan and cyclosporine), as well as supplements.

- If you have an aortic stenosis, because you should not take amlodipine.
- If you have liver disease.
- If you plan to have surgery, including dental surgery, tell your doctor or dentist you are taking amlodipine.

Of Special Interest to Women
- Amlodipine should not be taken during pregnancy unless your doctor decides it is necessary. Discuss the benefits and risks.
- It is not known if amlodipine passes into breast milk. Talk to your doctor before you breast-feed.

Symptoms of Overdose
Fainting, light-headedness, and rapid heartbeat.

Amoxicillin

Brand Name
Amoxil
Available as Generic?
Yes
Principal Uses
Various bacterial infections, including but not limited to bronchitis, chlamydia, cystitis, gonorrhea, Lyme disease, middle ear infections, urinary tract infections
About the Drug
Amoxicillin is a penicillin. Other antibiotics in this group are ampicillin (Unasyn), piperacillin (Pipracil), and ticarcillin (Ticar). Amoxicillin and other antibiotics in this group do not kill bacteria; instead, they prevent bacteria from multiplying by stopping the formation of walls that surround and protect them. Amoxicillin is effective against various bacteria, including *H. influenzae, N. gonorrhoeae, E. coli, Pneumococci, Streptococci,* and certain strains of *Staphylococci.*
How to Use This Drug
Amoxicillin is available as capsules, tablets, extended-release tablets, chewable tablets, and oral suspension. The typical dose depends on the infections and can range from 250–500 mg every 8 hours, 500–875 mg every 12 hours. For gonorrhea, 3 g are given as one dose. The tablets for oral suspension should not be swallowed whole or chewed; mix them with 2 teaspoons of water and swallow. Swallow the extended-release tablets whole; do not chew or crush them.

The antibiotic can be taken with or without food. Drink lots of fluids while you are taking amoxicillin unless your health-care provider tells you otherwise. Because antibiotics work best if you maintain a steady level of the medication in your body, make sure to take your doses at the same time each day. Do not stop taking your prescription before the entire treatment course is done, even if you feel better, because the infection may return if you do.

Side Effects

- Common side effects: abdominal pain, allergic reactions, confusion, diarrhea, dizziness, heartburn, insomnia, itching, nausea, rash, and vomiting.
- Unlikely but serious side effects that should be reported to your health-care provider immediately: dark urine, easy bruising or bleeding, persistent fever or sore throat, persistent nausea or vomiting, stomach pain, and yellowing of the eyes or skin.
- Rarely, amoxicillin causes *Clostridium difficile*–associated diarrhea, which may occur weeks to months after treatment has stopped. Symptoms may include abdominal pain or cramping, blood or mucus in the stool, and persistent diarrhea.
- Prolonged use of amoxicillin may cause oral thrush or a new vaginal yeast infection.

Possible Drug, Supplement, and/or Food Interactions

- Probenecid slows the removal of amoxicillin from your body.
- Amoxicillin may reduce the effectiveness of combination-type birth control pills.

Tell Your Doctor

- If you have any allergies and all OTC and prescription medications you are taking, as well as supplements.
- If you have kidney disease or infectious mononucleosis.
- If you are taking methotrexate or tetracyclines, or if you plan to get a live bacterial vaccine (e.g., BCG for tuberculosis).
- Tell your doctor and lab personnel you are taking amoxicillin before you undergo lab tests, because the antibiotic may affect the results.

Of Special Interest to Women

- Although penicillins are generally considered safe during pregnancy, consult your health-care provider before taking amoxicillin if you are pregnant. He or she should make sure you are not allergic to penicillin.
- Amoxicillin passes into breast milk and may cause diarrhea or allergic

responses in nursing infants. However, amoxicillin is generally considered safe while breast-feeding, as this antibiotic is prescribed to treat infections in newborns. Consult your health-care provider before you breast-feed.

Symptoms of Overdose

Persistent diarrhea, seizures, severe vomiting, and a severe decrease in the amount of urine.

Anastrozole

Brand Name

Arimidex

Available as Generic?

Yes

Principal Use

Breast cancer

About the Drug

Anastrozole is a nonsteroidal aromatase inhibitor. Letrozole (Femara) is also in this drug category. Anastrozole works by lowering the amount of estrogen the body produces in an attempt to shrink breast tumors and slow their growth.

Anastrozole is used alone or with other treatments, such as radiation therapy or surgery, to treat early breast cancer in women who have gone through menopause. It is also used to treat breast cancer in women whose cancer has worsened after they have taken tamoxifen, and by women (after menopause) as a first treatment of breast cancer that has metastasized (spread) within the breast or to other areas of the body. Occasionally it is prescribed to prevent breast cancer in women who are at high risk of the disease.

How to Use This Drug

Anastrozole is available in tablets and can be taken with or without food. It is usually taken once daily, and it should be taken at the same time each day. Some women need to take anastrozole for years. Continue to take this medication even if you feel well. Do not stop taking anastrozole without consulting your doctor.

Side Effects

- Most common side effects: body aches and pains, breast swelling or tenderness, constipation, diarrhea, dizziness, dry mouth, hair thinning, hot flashes, increased cough, loss of appetite, nausea, scratchy throat, trouble sleeping, tiredness/weakness, vaginal bleeding, and vomiting.

- Less common but serious side effects: bone fracture, bone pain, chills, depression, fever, numbness, tingling or swelling of the hands or feet, persistent cough, unusually stiff muscles, unusual vaginal discharge, vaginal burning or itching, and vision changes.
- Rare but serious side effects: breathing difficulties, chest pain, confusion, fainting, jaw and/or left arm pain, slurred speech, and weakness on one side of the body.

Possible Drug, Supplement, and/or Food Interactions

- Do not use alcohol while taking anastrozole.
- Anastrozole should never be used with estrogens (e.g., hormone replacement therapy or hormonal contraceptives such as birth control pills, patches, rings, or injections), raloxifene, or tamoxifen because very serious interactions may occur.

Tell Your Doctor

- If you have any allergies, and all prescription and OTC medications you are taking, as well as supplements.
- If you have liver disease, high blood pressure, heart disease, osteoporosis, or blood clots.

Of Special Interest to Women

- Because anastrozole can be absorbed through the skin, women who are pregnant or who may become pregnant should not handle or break the tablets.
- Anastrozole can decrease bone density and thus may cause or worsen osteoporosis. It may also increase the risk of fracture.
- Although anastrozole is usually prescribed for women who have gone through menopause, if you become pregnant or think you may be pregnant, tell your doctor immediately.
- Anastrozole should not be used if you are breast-feeding because of potential risk to the infant.

Symptoms of Overdose

Not known.

Aripiprazole

Brand Name

Abilify

Available as Generic?

No

Principal Uses

Bipolar disorder, major depression, schizophrenia

About the Drug

Aripiprazole is a second-generation, or atypical antipsychotic. Other drugs in this category include clozapine (Clozaril), olanzapine (Zyprexa), quetiapine (Seroquel), risperidone (Risperdal), and ziprasidone (Geodon).

Experts are not certain how aripiprazole works. However, aripiprazole is known to block or reduce the effects of several chemicals in the brain (including dopamine and serotonin) that are often elevated in people who have schizophrenia or bipolar disorder. Aripiprazole is also used to treat major depression in individuals who have not responded well to antidepressants. Therefore, aripiprazole is typically added to an antidepressant treatment program, and this has been found to significantly reduce depression symptoms when compared with placebo.

How to Use This Drug

Aripiprazole is available in regular tablets, rapidly dissolving tablets (Abilify Discmelt), and liquid form for those who have difficulty swallowing pills. Dosing is typically once daily with a starting dose of 10–15 mg, which can be increased over time. You should take aripiprazole at the same time each day. The drug can be taken with or without food, but if you experience stomach irritation, take it with food.

If you are using the rapidly dissolving tablets, make sure your hands are dry when you handle the tablet. Place the tablet under your tongue and allow it to dissolve: Do not chew, crush, or break the tablet. No water is needed, as you can swallow the dissolved pill with saliva.

Side Effects

- Most common side effects: anxiety, blurry vision, constipation, cough, headache, insomnia, light-headedness, nausea, rash, restlessness, runny nose, sleepiness, vomiting, weakness, and weight gain.
- Unlikely but serious side effects, which should be reported immediately to your doctor: fast/pounding heartbeat, fainting, mood changes (e.g., suicidal thoughts, depression), weakness, tremors, trouble swallowing, swelling of the ankles and/or feet, seizures, and signs of infection.
- Long-term use of aripiprazole may cause a potentially irreversible condition called tardive dyskinesia, characterized by involuntary movements of the jaw, lips, and tongue. A potentially fatal condition

called neuroleptic malignant syndrome has been reported with antipsychotic drugs, including aripiprazole. This condition is characterized by excessive sweating, heart arrhythmias, altered mental state, irregular pulse, rapid heart rate, high fever, and muscle rigidity.

- Individuals who take aripiprazole should be tested for elevated blood sugar levels both before and while taking the drug, especially those who have risk factors for diabetes, such as obesity or a family history of diabetes.
- There is a slight increased risk of heart failure, pneumonia, and stroke when this medication is taken by elderly patients who have dementia.
- Aripiprazole can increase your risk of developing heat stroke, so be careful not to overheat.

Possible Drug, Supplement, and/or Food Interactions

- Several drugs can increase the rate at which the body's enzymes degrade aripiprazole, which in turn can significantly decrease the amount of aripiprazole in the body: carbamazepine (Tegretol), phenytoin (Dilantin), rifampin (Rifadin), and phenobarbitol.
- Other drugs are either known to or have the potential to block CYP3A4, a liver enzyme that degrades aripiprazole: ketoconazole (Nizoral; known to block the enzyme), itraconazole (Sporanox), fluconazole (Diflucan), voriconazole (Vfend), cimetidine (Tagamet), verapamil (Calan), diltiazem (Cardizem), erythromycin, clarithromycin (Biaxin), nefazodone (Serzone), and indinavir (Crixivan).
- Do not drink grapefruit juice or eat grapefruit while you take aripiprazole.
- Quinidine, fluoxetine (Prozac), and paroxetine (Paxil) inhibit the liver enzyme CYP2D6, which also breaks down aripiprazole and can increase the level of aripiprazole in the body.
- Alpha-1 receptor blockers, such as doxazosin (Cardura), prazosin (Minipres), and terazosin (Hytrin), may seriously lower blood pressure if taken with aripiprazole.
- Some drugs may increase the risk of seizures when combined with aripiprazole, such as bupropion, isoniazid, phenothiazines, theophylline, tramadol, and tricyclic antidepressants (e.g., amitriptyline).
- Other drugs that may cause an undesirable interaction include dopamine agonists (e.g., bromocriptine), blood pressure medication, levodopa, antihistamines, medications for sleep or anxiety (e.g., alprazolam, diazepam), muscle relaxants, narcotic pain relievers (e.g., codeine), and psychiatric medications (e.g., risperidone, trazodone).

Tell Your Doctor

- If you have a history of cerebrovascular disease, stroke, dehydration, diabetes, heart problems, nervous system problems (e.g., dementia, seizures), obesity, trouble swallowing, alcohol and/or drug abuse, and low white blood cell count.
- About any prescription and all OTC medications or supplements you are taking, as well as allergies.
- If you have diabetes, as the liquid medication may contain sugar and you should take the tablets instead.
- If you have phenylketonuria or any other condition that requires you to restrict your intake of phenylalanine or aspartame, as the rapidly dissolving tablets may contain aspartame.

Of Special Interest to Women

- Aripiprazole has not been studied in pregnant women, but some undesirable effects have been observed in animal studies. Your doctor may decide to prescribe aripiprazole if he or she believes its benefits outweigh potential risks.
- Experts do not know if aripiprazole is excreted in breast milk. However, because many medications are, generally women who take aripiprazole should not breast-feed.

Symptoms of Overdose

Loss of consciousness and very rapid heartbeat.

Azathioprine

Brand Names

Imuran, Azasan

Available as Generic?

Yes

Principal Uses

Severe rheumatoid arthritis in patients who do not respond to NSAIDs, and to prevent rejection of a kidney transplant; off-label use includes multiple sclerosis, Crohn's disease, myasthenia gravis, chronic ulcerative colitis, autoimmune hepatitis

About the Drug

Azathioprine is an immunosuppressive, which means it suppresses the activity of the immune system. In the body, azathioprine is converted into its active form, called mercaptopurine. Azathioprine works by suppressing the spread of white blood cells called T and B lymphocytes, which defend the body against infectious diseases and foreign invaders. If you have rheumatoid arthritis, for example, azathioprine could blunt your immune system, which in turn would reduce the inflammation associated with immune reactions and also slow damage to your joints caused by the inflammation.

How to Use This Drug

Azathioprine is available in tablets. You can take azathioprine with food to reduce the chance of stomach upset. For treating rheumatoid arthritis, a common dose does not exceed 2.5 mg per kilogram per day. It may take up to 2 months of continued use before you notice symptom relief. If you don't experience improvement after taking azathioprine for 3 months, contact your doctor.

Side Effects

- Most common serious side effects: severe lowering of the white blood cell count, which can result in an increased risk of infections; and gastrointestinal effects, including nausea, vomiting, and loss of appetite. If these symptoms persist, contact your physician immediately.
- Less frequent side effects: diarrhea, fatigue, hair loss, and joint pain.
- Prolonged use of azathioprine may increase your risk of developing certain types of cancer (e.g., lymphoma, skin cancer).
- In rare cases, azathioprine can cause serious (or fatal) blood disorders. This risk is greater in patients who take azathioprine to prevent kidney transplant rejection than in those who take it for rheumatoid arthritis.
- Contact your health-care provider immediately if you experience any of the following: change in the appearance or size of moles, difficulty swallowing, easy bruising or bleeding, mouth sores, muscle loss, night sweats, signs of infection (e.g., fever, persistent sore throat), unusual growths or lumps, unusual tiredness, vision changes, and yellowing of the skin or eyes.

Possible Drug, Supplement, and/or Food Interactions

- Allopurinol increases levels of azathioprine in the body and may also increase the risk of side effects from azathioprine.
- ACE inhibitors (e.g., lisinopril) may cause anemia and severe leucopenia if taken with azathioprine.
- Azathioprine may reduce the ability of warfarin to thin the blood.

- Azathioprine used with the following medications can result in very serious interactions: chlorambucil, cyclophosphamide, febuxostat, melphalan, mercaptopurine, natalizumab.

Tell Your Doctor
- If you have any allergies and all prescription and OTC medications you are taking, as well as supplements.
- If you have kidney disease, liver disease, blood disorders, cancer, active infections, decreased bone marrow function, or the enzyme disorder TPMT deficiency.
- Before you get any type of immunization/vaccination, and avoid contact with anyone who has recently received an oral polio vaccine or intranasal flu vaccine.

Of Special Interest to Women
- Azathioprine is known to harm the fetus, so avoid this drug if you are pregnant or are planning to get pregnant.
- Azathioprine is passed into breast milk. Consult your doctor before breast-feeding.
- Azathioprine can be absorbed through the skin, so if you are pregnant or planning to get pregnant, do not handle or break the tablets.

Symptoms of Overdose
Not known.

Azithromycin

Brand Names
Zithromax, Zmax

Available as Generic?
Yes

Principal Uses
Infections caused by various bacteria, such as *Hemophilus influenzae, Streptococcus pneumoniae, Mycoplasma pneumoniae,* and *Staphylococcus aureus.* These may include bronchitis, laryngitis, otitis media (middle ear infection), pelvic inflammatory disease, pneumonia, sinusitis, tonsillitis, and several sexually transmitted infectious diseases such as cervicitis, chlamydia, and nongonococcal urethritis

About the Drug
Azithromycin is a semisynthetic macrolide antibiotic that was the fifth most popular drug in the United States in 2009, with 53 million pre-

scriptions written, according to an IMS health report. Other drugs in the macrolide group include clarithromycin (Biaxin), erythromycin, and telithromycin (Ketek).

Azithromycin, like other antibiotics in its drug class, prevents the growth of bacteria by interfering with their ability to make proteins. An advantage of azithromycin over many other antibiotics is that it has a long half-life, which means it stays in the body for quite a long time. This allows patients to take it only once a day and for a shorter period of time for most infections. Azithromycin is not effective against viruses (e.g., common cold, flu).

How to Use This Drug

Azithromycin is available in tablets and suspension for patient use and in powder for hospital use via injection. The drug can be taken with or without food, but food can reduce the chance of stomach upset. Take Zmax, the oral suspension, extended-release form, on an empty stomach 1 hour before or 2 hours after a meal, because food reduces the body's ability to absorb the drug.

The adult dose of azithromycin is 500–2000 mg in 1 or divided doses, although Zmax is usually given as a single 2000 mg dose. Your first dose will likely be a double dose, twice as much as the remainder of the doses you will need to take. Azithromycin is usually taken for 3–5 days, and it should be taken at the same time each day for optimal effectiveness.

Side Effects

- Most common side effects: abdominal pain, diarrhea or loose stools, nausea, and vomiting. These occur in less than 5% of patients.
- Rare side effects: abnormal liver test results, allergic reactions, and nervousness.
- Contact your doctor immediately if you experience any of these rare but serious side effects: hearing loss, blurry vision, slurred speech, dark urine, persistent nausea/vomiting, severe stomach pain, yellowing of the eyes or skin, dizziness, fainting, irregular heartbeat, or muscle weakness.
- In rare cases, a serious condition called *Clostridium difficile*–associated diarrhea, which is caused by a type of resistant bacteria, may occur during treatment or even weeks to months after treatment has ended.

Possible Drug, Supplement, and/or Food Interactions

- Azithromycin (except Zmax) should not be taken at the same time as aluminum- or magnesium-based antacids, because the antacids will prevent the antibiotic from being absorbed. There should be at least a 2-hour gap between the time you take these antacids and when you take azithromycin.

- Azithromycin with antiarrhythmic drugs (e.g., amiodarone, disopyramide, dofetilide, quinidine, procainamide, sotalol) and certain quinolones, such as gatifloxacin, grepafloxacin, and moxifloxacin, may increase the risk of ventricular arrhythmias including torsade de pointes and sudden death.
- Warfarin with azithromycin may increase your risk of bleeding.
- Azithromycin with any of the following drugs may increase the levels of the drugs in the body: carbamazepine, cyclosporine, digoxin, ergot alkaloids, phenytoin, quinine, tacrolimus, theopylline, triazolam.
- Nelfinavir may raise the levels of azithromycin in the body.

Tell Your Doctor

- About any allergies, especially to other macrolide antibiotics such as clarithromycin or erythromycin, or to ketolide antibiotics such as telithromycin.
- About all prescription and OTC medications you are taking, as well as supplements.
- If you have a history of liver disease, kidney disease, myasthenia gravis, heart failure, slow heartbeat, or QT prolongation in the EKG; or a family history of QT prolongation in the EKG or sudden cardiac death.
- If you take diuretics, if you have low levels of magnesium or potassium, and/or if you experience severe sweating, diarrhea, or vomiting, all of which may increase your risk of QT prolongation.

Of Special Interest to Women

- Take azithromycin during pregnancy only if your doctor deems it is necessary. No adequate tests have been done to determine if it is safe for pregnant women.
- It is not known whether azithromycin is secreted in breast milk. Discuss the benefits and risks associated with the use of azithromycin during breast-feeding with your health-care provider.
- Prolonged or repeated use of azithromycin may result in a vaginal yeast infection or oral thrush. Contact your physician if you notice a change in vaginal discharge or other symptoms, or if you develop white patches in your mouth, which are signs of thrush.

Symptoms of Overdose

Diarrhea, nausea and vomiting, and loss of strength.

Black Cohosh

Brand Names

Various brands over-the-counter, including Eclectic Institute, Gaia Herbs, Nature's Way

Principal Uses

Symptoms of menopause, premenstrual syndrome, arthritis

About the Herb

Black cohosh (*Actaea racemosa;* formerly *Cimicifuga racemosa*), which is also known as black snakeroot, bugbane, and rattleroot, is a tall flowering plant indigenous to the northeastern part of the United States. It was used by Native Americans more than two centuries ago for many of the same indications for which women use it today. The herb has been highly researched; it is an approved remedy in Germany for premenstrual, menstrual, and menopausal symptoms, and it is widely used throughout Europe.

Black cohosh contains sugar compounds (glycosides), isoferulic acids (which have anti-inflammatory properties), and possibly phytoestrogens (plant-based estrogens). The possibility that black cohosh has estrogenlike activity has been studied, but the results are contradictory. The herb may also have an impact on luteinizing hormone and follicle-stimulating hormone, but here as well the study results do not agree. Numerous clinical studies confirm that black cohosh is effective for improving menopausal symptoms, including hot flashes, night sweats, vaginal dryness, including some evidence from a 2007 study published in *Advances in Therapy* that black cohosh is more effective than fluoxetine (Prozac) in relieving these symptoms.

How to Use This Herb

Black cohosh is available in capsules, tablets, liquid tincture, extracts, and dried root for tea. The suggested dose is 40–80 mg daily of tablets or capsules standardized to contain 1 mg of 27-deoxyactein. For tinctures, 2–4 mL 3 times daily is recommended. Teas typically are not as effective as a standardized extract. To make a black cohosh tea, bring to a boil 2 grams of dried root and 34 ounces of water, and then simmer for 20–30 minutes until the liquid is reduced by one-third. Drink 1 cup 3 times daily. Black cohosh is also available in combination formulas, often with dong quai, licorice, and/or red clover.

Side Effects
- At recommended doses, side effects are generally mild and may include abdominal discomfort, headache, and rash.
- At high doses, side effects may include abdominal pain, diarrhea, dizziness, headache, joint pain, nausea, slow heart rate, tremors, vision problems, vomiting, and weight gain.

Possible Drug, Supplement, and/or Food Interactions
- Black cohosh may affect how your body handles certain antidepressants (e.g., amitriptyline, desipramine, imipramine, paroxetine, venlafaxine) as well as codeine, flecainide, haloperidol, metoprolol, risperidone, and tramadol. Avoid taking black cohosh with any of these drugs.
- Black cohosh may make cisplatin less effective in the treatment of breast cancer.

Tell Your Doctor
- About any allergies you have, and all prescription or OTC medications you are taking, as well as supplements.
- If you have a history of breast cancer or have a high risk for developing breast cancer.
- If you have a liver disorder or if you develop symptoms such as abdominal pain, jaundice, or dark urine while taking black cohosh. Hepatitis (inflamed liver) and liver failure have been seen in several women who used black cohosh, although it is not certain the herb was responsible.

Of Special Interest to Women
- The American College of Obstetricians and Gynecologists recognizes the value of black cohosh for treatment of menopausal symptoms. Some doctors, however, recommend using black cohosh for only 6 months or less because not enough is known about the long-term effects of the herb.
- Studies of black cohosh have yielded controversial results. A Yale study reported that black cohosh may interfere with radiation and chemotherapy drugs given for breast cancer. The possibility that black cohosh may contain phytoestrogens, which can stimulate the growth of breast tumors, has raised some questions about its use in women. The most recent (2010) findings on this topic come from the VITAL (VITamins And Lifestyle) Cohort, in which more than 35,000 postmenopausal women participated. The investigators did not find any increased risk of breast cancer associated with the use of black co-

hosh. (No increased risk was found for soy, Saint-John's-wort, or dong quai either.) Even so, women who have breast cancer, a history of breast cancer, or risk factors for the disease should talk to their doctor before taking black cohosh.

- Numerous animal studies have suggested that black cohosh may help prevent bone loss and thus osteoporosis. However, more research is needed, especially in humans, to support these preliminary findings.
- Women who are pregnant or breast-feeding should not take black cohosh. In pregnant women, it may stimulate contractions and lead to premature labor.
- Black cohosh should not be confused with blue cohosh (*Caulophyllum thalictroides*), which is an entirely different herb with different properties, side effects, and uses. Although black cohosh has been used along with blue cohosh to stimulate labor, this combination has caused adverse effects in newborns, and these negative effects appear to be due to blue cohosh.

Symptoms of Overdose

Dizziness, nausea, vomiting, excessive perspiration, reduced pulse rate, and nervous system disturbances. One case of convulsions has been documented.

Calcium

Brand Names

Various brands over-the-counter, including Caltrate, Citracal, Nature Made

Available as Generic?

Yes

Principal Uses

Prevention and treatment of bone loss/osteoporosis

About the Supplement

Calcium is the most abundant mineral in the body. It is found naturally in a variety of foods and added to others, but our focus here is the supplement form. Calcium supplements are taken to prevent or treat low calcium levels in people who do not get a sufficient amount of calcium from their diet. Calcium supplements are commonly taken by women (and men) to treat bone loss, weak bones (osteomalacia), and decreased activity of the parathyroid gland. They are also taken by women who are pregnant, nursing, or postmenopausal, as well as by individuals who are using certain medications (e.g., phenytoin, phenobarbital, prednisone), which decrease the amount of calcium available to the body. (See, however, "Of Special Interest to Women" below regarding a new warning about calcium supplements.)

Ninety-nine percent of the calcium in the body is stored in the bones and teeth, where it is necessary for the continued health and maintenance of these structures. Among aging adults, especially postmenopausal women, a decline in calcium absorption and the breakdown of bone progresses faster than bone formation, which results in bone loss and the risk of osteoporosis.

The remaining 1% of calcium in the body is in the blood, muscle, and intercellular fluids, where it is necessary for muscle contraction, the secretion of hormones and enzymes, transmitting signals in the nervous system, and blood vessel health.

How to Use This Supplement

Calcium supplements are available in tablets, capsules, liquid, chewable "candies," and powder. These supplements can be taken with or without food, depending on the form (e.g., calcium carbonate, calcium citrate, etc.). Your body cannot absorb more than 600 mg of calcium at one time. So, for example, if your doctor has recommended you take 800 mg of calcium per day, take 400 mg twice a day.

Vitamin D helps the body better absorb calcium, so talk to your doctor about getting enough of this important vitamin as well, either through regular but limited exposure to sunlight, vitamin D–rich foods, and/or supplementation. Calcium supplements are often available in a combination form, most often with vitamin D and/or magnesium. Talk to your health-care provider about the optimal supplement for your specific needs.

The National Academy of Sciences states that the recommended daily allowance of calcium for women is 1000 mg for those age 19–50 regardless of whether they are pregnant or breast-feeding; and 1200 mg for those 51 and older. Women between the ages of 9 and 18 need 1300 mg whether or not they are pregnant or breast-feeding.

The two main forms of calcium supplements are carbonate and citrate; others include gluconate, lactate, and phosphate. Calcium carbonate is more readily available and inexpensive than calcium citrate. Both carbonate and citrate forms are absorbed similarly, but people who have low levels of stomach acid can absorb calcium citrate more easily. The body absorbs calcium carbonate more efficiently if the supplement is taken with food, although the body can absorb calcium citrate equally well with or without food.

Side Effects

- Common side effects: constipation and upset stomach.
- Rare side effects: bone or muscle pain, headache, increased thirst and/ or urination, loss of appetite, mood changes, nausea, unusual tiredness, and vomiting.

Possible Drug, Supplement, and/or Food Interactions

- Calcium can decrease the absorption of certain drugs. It is recommended that you take bisphosphonates (e.g., alendronate) at least 30 minutes before taking calcium. When using tetracycline antibiotics, take calcium at least 2 hours before or 4 hours after the drugs. With quinolone antibiotics (e.g., ciprofloxacin), take calcium at least 1 hour after. For levothyroxine, take calcium at least 4 hours before or after the drug dose.
- Thiazide-type diuretics can interact with calcium carbonate supplements and increase your risk of hypercalcemia (abnormally high calcium in the blood) and hypercalciuria (abnormally high levels of calcium in the urine), two potentially serious conditions.
- Antacids that contain aluminum or magnesium increase excretion of calcium in the urine.
- Mineral oil and stimulant laxatives decrease the body's ability to absorb calcium.
- Glucocorticoids, such as prednisone, can deplete calcium from the body and eventually result in osteoporosis if they are taken for months.
- Calcium may interact with digoxin, cellulose sodium phosphate, and certain phosphate binders (e.g., calcium acetate), so talk to your doctor before starting calcium supplementation if you take any of these products.
- Intravenous ceftriaxone and calcium can cause life-threatening damage to the kidneys and lungs. These two substances should not be given intravenously within 48 hours of each other.
- Estrogen helps your body absorb calcium. Therefore, taking estrogen along with large amounts of calcium may raise the level of calcium in the blood to unhealthy levels.

Tell Your Doctor

- About any allergies you have, and all prescription and OTC medications you are taking, as well as supplements.

- If you have kidney disease, kidney stones, little or no stomach acid (achlorhydria), heart disease, disease of the pancreas, sarcoidosis, difficulty absorbing nutrition from food, or high levels of calcium.
- If you are pregnant or breast-feeding.

Of Special Interest to Women

Because so many women rely on calcium supplements to help prevent osteoporosis or while pregnant or breast-feeding, it is important to know that a recent meta-analysis published in the *British Journal of Medicine* reported a 30% increased risk of heart attack among older adults who took calcium supplements. Authors of the study pointed out that when you take calcium supplements, the level of calcium in the blood rises over the following 4–6 hours and climbs to the top limit of normal.

These high levels of calcium in the blood can lead to the development of plaques in the blood vessels, which in turn can result in heart attack, stroke, and other cardiovascular diseases. This rise in blood calcium levels does not happen when you eat foods rich in calcium because the body absorbs the mineral slowly, so blood calcium levels hardly fluctuate at all. Therefore, you may want to reconsider how to get the calcium your body needs for bone health.

Symptoms of Overdose

Nausea and vomiting, loss of appetite, headache, unusual tiredness, weakness, and mental/mood changes.

Celecoxib

Brand Name
Celebrex

Available as Generic?
No

Principal Uses
Pain, fever, swelling, and tenderness associated with osteoarthritis, rheumatoid arthritis, and ankylosing spondylitis; also menstrual cramps, colonic polyps associated with familial adenomatous polyposis

About the Drug
Celecoxib is an NSAID that works by blocking the enzyme that produces prostaglandins (cyclooxygenase 2, or COX-2), which results in lower production of COX-2. Prostaglandins are chemicals that contribute to inflammation in arthritis, which results in pain, fever, tenderness, and swelling. Celecoxib differs from other NSAIDs because it is less likely to

cause inflammation and ulceration of the stomach and intestinal tract with short-term use, and does not hamper the clotting of blood. Other commonly used NSAIDs include diclofenac (Voltaren), ibuprofen (Motrin), indomethacin (Indocin), ketoprofen (Orudis), naproxen (Aleve), piroxicam (Feldene), and sulindac (Clinoril).

Celecoxib also is helpful in reducing the cramping and pain associated with menstruation, symptoms that are due to prostaglandins. Individuals who have familial adenomatous polyposis are also treated with celecoxib, as the drug helps prevent the formation and reduces the size of polyps that develop in large numbers in the colon.

For certain conditions, such as arthritis, it may take up to 2 weeks of regular use before you notice significant benefits from celecoxib. If you take celecoxib on an as-needed basis, you will likely get your best results if you take the drug when the first signs of pain occur rather than when the pain has advanced.

How to Use This Drug

Celecoxib is available in capsules. The typical dose for osteoarthritis is 100 mg twice daily or 200 mg once. For rheumatoid arthritis, the dose is usually 100 or 200 mg twice daily. For acute pain or menstrual cramps, the typical dose is 400 mg as a single dose on the first day of symptoms, followed by an additional 200 mg as needed, then 200 mg twice daily as needed. For familial adenomatous polyposis, the typical dose is 400 mg twice daily. You should always strive to take the lowest effective dose.

To reduce the risk of stomach upset, you can take celecoxib with food. Take celecoxib with 8 ounces of water unless your doctor tells you otherwise. After taking celecoxib, do not lie down for at least 30 minutes.

Side Effects

- Common side effects: constipation, diarrhea, dizziness, gas, headache, heartburn, nausea, sore throat, stomach upset, and stuffy nose.
- Seek medical attention immediately if these less common, severe side effects occur: severe allergic reactions (e.g., breathing difficulties; hives; itching; rash; swelling of the mouth, face, lips, or tongue), bloody or black tarry stools, change in urination volume, dark urine, chest pain, confusion, depression, fainting, fast or irregular heartbeat, fever, chills, hearing loss, mental or mood changes, numbness in an arm or leg, skin changes (e.g., swollen, blistered, peeling), ringing in the ears, seizures, severe stomach pain or nausea, severe vomiting, unusual joint or muscle pain, unusual tiredness or weakness, vision or speech problems, yellowing of the eyes or skin.

- Celecoxib rarely causes serious liver disease. Indications of liver disease include yellowing of the eyes or skin, dark urine, persistent abdominal pain, and unusual fatigue.
- NSAIDs, including celecoxib, may increase the risk of heart attack, stroke, and related conditions, which can be fatal. This risk may be greater if you have risk factors for heart and blood vessel conditions, and the longer you use celecoxib.

Possible Drug, Supplement, and/or Food Interactions

- Celecoxib along with aspirin or other NSAIDs may increase the occurrence of gastrointestinal ulcers and other side effects. Check the labels of all prescription and OTC medications you are taking to make sure they do not include NSAIDs.
- Celecoxib with cidofovir can result in very serious interactions.
- Celecoxib may interact with the following drugs, so inform your doctor or pharmacist before starting celecoxib: antiplatelet drugs (e.g., cilostazol, clopidogrel), ACE inhibitors (e.g., captopril), angiotensin II receptor blockers (e.g., losartan), bisphosphonates (e.g., alendronate), blood thinners (e.g., warfarin, heparin), corticosteroids (e.g., prednisone), desmopressin, diuretics (e.g., furosemide).
- Celecoxib with aspirin or other NSAIDs, such as ibuprofen and naproxen, may increase the development of stomach and intestinal ulcers.
- Fluconazole increases the concentration of celecoxib in the body. Your doctor may prescribe celecoxib at the lowest recommended dose if you are also taking fluconazole.
- Celecoxib increases the concentration of lithium in the blood and may result in side effects. Therefore, your doctor should monitor your lithium therapy closely during and after treatment with celecoxib.

Tell Your Doctor

- If you are allergic to aspirin or other NSAIDs, or if you have other allergies, as well as all prescription and OTC medications you use, along with supplements.
- If you have aspirin-sensitive asthma.
- If you have had recent heart bypass surgery.
- About any history of stroke or other cerebrovascular disease, kidney problems, liver problems, heart disease, alcohol use, blood disorders (e.g., anemia), serious infections, asthma, swelling, bleeding or clotting problems, gastrointestinal problems, dehydration, poorly controlled diabetes, or growths in the nose.

Of Special Interest to Women
- Celecoxib should be used only when prescribed by a physician during the first six months of pregnancy and never taken during the last three months. Studies show there is a risk of heart defects in the newborn when celecoxib is taken in late pregnancy.
- Celecoxib passes into breast milk. Although there have not been any reports of harm to nursing infants, consult your doctor before breast-feeding.
- Although use of celecoxib and aspirin together may increase your risk of side effects, if your doctor has prescribed low doses of aspirin to prevent heart attack or stroke, he or she will likely ask you to continue to take the aspirin. Discuss any concerns with your physician.

Symptoms of Overdose
Severe stomach pain, coffee ground–like vomit, change in the amount of urine produced, shallow or slow breathing, severe headache, or loss of consciousness.

Cephalexin

Brand Name
Keflex
Available as Generic?
Yes
Principal Uses
A variety of bacterial infections, including urinary tract infections; skin infections; bone infections; pneumonia; bronchitis; and infections that affect the middle ear, tonsils, throat, and larynx
About the Drug
Cephalexin is a cephalosporin. Drugs in this class (e.g., cefaclor, cefadroxil, cefdinir, cefditoren, cefixime, cefprozil, ceftazidime, and cefuroxime) are similar to penicillin in side effects and in how they work to treat bacterial infections: They prevent bacteria from developing cell walls around themselves; bacteria that cannot build these cell walls die. Bacteria that can be destroyed using cephalexin include *Staphylococcus aureus, Streptococcus pneumoniae, Haemophilus influenzae,* and *E. coli.*
How to Use This Drug
Cephalexin is available as tablets, capsules, and powder for suspension. The usual dosing schedule is 1–4 grams in divided doses every 6 or 12

hours, or as directed by your doctor. You can take cephalexin with food if the medication upsets your stomach. If you are using the suspension, shake the bottle well before using it. Use the measuring device provided with the prescription; do not use a household spoon.

Because antibiotics work best if the drug is kept at a constant level in your body, make sure to take cephalexin at evenly spaced intervals. Complete the entire course of treatment even if you feel better before the medication is done, because stopping too early can allow the infection to return.

Side Effects

- Common side effects: abnormal liver test results, diarrhea, dizziness, fever, headache, rash, stomach upset, vaginitis, and vomiting.
- Unlikely but very serious side effects that should be reported to your health-care provider immediately: change in the amount or color of urine, easy bruising or bleeding, flulike symptoms, mental/mood changes, persistent nausea/vomiting, severe abdominal pain, and yellowing of the skin or eyes.
- Abdominal pain/cramping, blood or mucus in your stool, and persistent diarrhea may indicate a severe intestinal condition called *Clostridium difficile*–associated diarrhea, which is caused by resistant bacteria. This condition can develop while you are taking cephalexin or weeks to months after you have stopped treatment. Contact your physician immediately if these symptoms occur.
- Long-term or repeated use of cephalexin may cause oral thrush (white patches in your mouth) or a new vaginal yeast infection.

Possible Drug, Supplement, and/or Food Interactions

- Cephalexin may reduce the effectiveness of combination birth control pills and result in pregnancy. You may need to use additional birth control protection while taking cephalexin.
- Cephalexin may interfere with the results of certain lab tests, such as Coombs' test and urine glucose tests. Be sure to tell your health-care provider and lab personnel you are taking cephalexin.
- Limit your use of alcohol while taking cephalexin.

Tell Your Doctor

- If you have any allergies, especially to cephalosporins or to penicillins, and also all OTC and prescription medications you are taking, as well as supplements.
- If you have kidney disease or stomach or intestinal disease.
- If you have diabetes, because the liquid form of this medication may contain sugar.

Of Special Interest to Women

- Cephalexin is an FDA pregnancy Category B medication, which means it is not expected to harm the fetus. However, do not take cephalexin during pregnancy without consulting your health-care provider about the benefits and risks.
- Cephalexin passes into breast milk and thus may harm a nursing infant. Tell your doctor if you are breast-feeding.

Symptoms of Overdose

Blood in the urine, persistent/severe vomiting, and seizures.

Ciprofloxacin

Brand Names

Cipro, Cipro XR, Proquin XR

Available as Generic?

Yes

Principal Uses

Infections of the skin, lungs, bones, and joints caused by bacteria; urinary tract infections, infectious diarrhea

About the Drug

Ciprofloxacin belongs to the fluoroquinolone class of antibiotics. This group includes gatifloxacin (Tequin), levofloxacin (Levaquin), moxifloxacin (Avelox), norfloxacin (Noroxin), ofloxacin (Floxin), and trovafloxacin (Trovan). Ciprofloxacin does not kill bacteria; it stops the multiplication of bacteria by disrupting the reproductive cycle and the ability of the bacteria to repair their genetic material.

How to Use This Drug

Ciprofloxacin is available in immediate-release tablets, extended-release tablets, microcapsules for suspension, and injection. The typical dose for most infections is 250–750 mg of the immediate-release tablets every 12 hours, or 500–1000 mg of the extended-release tablets every 24 hours. You can take the oral doses with or without food. However, there are certain foods and medications you should avoid or take only at certain times if you are using ciprofloxacin (see "Possible Drug, Supplement, and/or Food Interactions" below).

Take the entire course of ciprofloxacin as prescribed, even if you feel better before the prescription is done. Stopping early may allow bacteria to continue to grow and your infection to recur.

Side Effects

- Most common side effects: abdominal pain, diarrhea, headache, nausea, rash, restlessness, and vomiting.
- Unlikely but serious side effects that should be reported to your health-care provider immediately: changes in how you sense touch, pain, temperature, vibrations, or body position; change in urine color; confusion; fainting; fast or irregular heartbeat; hallucinations; mood/mental changes; mucus or blood in your stool; seizures; severe dizziness; severe/persistent headache; signs of a new infection; tremors; unusual bruising or bleeding; vision changes; and yellowing of the skin or eyes.
- Ciprofloxacin can change the normal bacteria in the colon and lead to the development of pseudomembranous colitis (an inflamed colon), which is characterized by abdominal pain, diarrhea, fever, and possibly shock.
- Chronic or repeated use of ciprofloxacin may cause oral thrush or a new vaginal yeast infection.
- Use of ciprofloxacin and other fluoroquinolones is associated with tendinitis and ruptured tendons, especially the Achilles' tendon. This risk is greatest if you are older than 60 or if you are taking corticosteroids (e.g., prednisone). In 2008, the FDA asked makers of fluoroquinolone antibiotics to add a black box warning to their drugs to warn consumers about the risk of spontaneous tendon ruptures and tendinitis from systemic use of these medications.
- In rare cases, ciprofloxacin can cause serious changes in blood sugar levels.

Possible Drug, Supplement, and/or Food Interactions

- Take ciprofloxacin at least 2 hours before or 6 hours after the following medications and supplements: quinapril; vitamins/minerals; iron and zinc supplements; products that contain aluminum, calcium, or magnesium (e.g., antacids, calcium supplements).
- Do not consume orange juice or calcium-rich foods within 6 hours before or 2 hours after taking ciprofloxacin unless they are part of a larger meal that contains other noncalcium foods.
- Ciprofloxacin can cause toxic levels of theophylline and result in seizures and heart rhythm disturbances.
- Ciprofloxacin may increase the blood-thinning effect of warfarin.
- Sevelamer may reduce the absorption of ciprofloxacin.

- Ciprofloxacin with strontium or tizanidine can result in very serious interactions.
- Ciprofloxacin with the following medications can increase the risk of heart rhythm disturbances: amiodarone, dofetilide, macrolide antibiotics (e.g., clarithromycin), quinidine, procainamide, sotalol, and some antipsychotic medications (e.g., thioridazine).
- Ciprofloxacin with isoniazid, phenothiazines, or tricyclic antidepressants (e.g., amitriptyline) may increase the risk of seizures.
- Ciprofloxacin may increase or prolong the effects of caffeine, so avoid consuming large amounts of beverages (e.g., colas, coffee), chocolate, or OTC products that contain caffeine.

Tell Your Doctor
- If you have any allergies, especially to any type of antibiotics, and all OTC and prescription medications you are taking, as well as supplements.
- If you have a central nervous system disease, such as seizures, or if you have diabetes, heart problems, joint or tendon problems, kidney disease, low levels of potassium or magnesium, or liver disease.

Of Special Interest to Women
- The safety of ciprofloxacin during pregnancy has not been established. Consult your health-care provider if you are pregnant or plan to get pregnant.
- Ciprofloxacin passes into breast milk. Since the safety of ciprofloxacin has not been established in nursing infants, you should not breast-feed while taking this medication.

Symptoms of Overdose
Diarrhea, slurred speech, and vomiting.

Cisplatin

Brand Name
Platinol-AQ
Available as Generic?
No
Principal Use
Chemotherapy for various types of cancer
About the Drug
Cisplatin is one of the main chemotherapy drugs used to treat cancer. It can be used alone or along with other medications to slow or stop

cancer cell growth. Cisplatin is a heavy metal (platinum) that destroys cells by disrupting their ability to multiply. It is commonly used to treat cancer of the ovaries, cervix, endometrium, bladder, head, and neck.

How to Use This Drug

Cisplatin is administered via injection into a vein (intravenously) by a health-care professional. The drug is usually given once every 3–4 weeks; the dose depends on your condition, body size, and how you respond to treatment.

While you are being treated with cisplatin, you should drink more fluids than usual, which will help you eliminate the drug more effectively and help avoid kidney side effects.

Side Effects

- Common side effects: diarrhea, loss of appetite, loss of taste, nausea, and vomiting. Temporary hair loss may also occur.
- Less likely but serious side effects you should report immediately to your health-care provider: black or bloody stools, blood in urine, change in the amount of urine, breathing difficulties, chest pain, confusion, dizziness, easy bruising or bleeding, fast heartbeat, hearing loss, jaw or left arm pain, loss of reflexes, loss of balance, lower back or side pain, nausea, numbness or tingling of the hands or feet, rash, seizures, signs of infection (e.g., fever, persistent sore throat), swelling of the face, and vision changes.
- Rarely, temporary loss of vision may occur; it usually returns after the end of treatment.

Possible Drug, Supplement, and/or Food Interactions

- Avoid contact with anyone who has recently received oral polio vaccine.
- Cisplatin with nalidixic acid or with pyridoxine combination with altretamine can cause very serious interactions.
- Cisplatin with etanercept, infliximab, and similar medications can increase the risk of infections.
- Cisplatin with clozapine may result in a significant decline in white blood cell count.
- Cisplatin with amiodarone, droperidol, and similar medications can increase the risk of heart arrhythmias and sudden death.

Tell Your Doctor

- If you have any allergies, especially to carboplatin, and all OTC and prescription medications you take, as well as supplements.

- If you have kidney disease, hearing problems, or decreased bone marrow function or blood cell disorders, as you should not take cisplatin.
- If you have gout, kidney stones, numbness or tingling of your hands or feet, or a mineral imbalance (low levels of calcium, magnesium, phosphate, potassium).
- Before you get any type of immunization or vaccination while you are being treated with cisplatin.

Of Special Interest to Women
- Cisplatin is not recommended during pregnancy, because it may harm the fetus.
- If you are of childbearing age, use reliable birth control methods during treatment with cisplatin and for at least 2–3 months after stopping treatment. Discuss with your doctor.
- Cisplatin passes into breast milk and poses potential harm to nursing infants. Use of this drug while breast-feeding is not recommended.
- Cisplatin can affect your ability to get pregnant after you have finished treatment. Discuss fertility with your doctor before you begin taking cisplatin.

Symptoms of Overdose
Extremely severe nausea and vomiting, kidney failure, liver failure, deafness, and even death.

Clomiphene Citrate

Brand Names
Clomid, Serophene
Available as Generic?
No
Principal Use
Female infertility
About the Drug
Clomiphene citrate is an antiestrogen drug in a class known as selective estrogen receptor modulators, or SERMs. It is often the first choice for treating infertility because it has a long history (25-plus years) of effective use. The drug causes the hypothalamus to release gonadotropin-releasing hormone, and the pituitary gland to release follicle-stimulating hormones and luteinizing hormones, which should trigger ovulation.

Clomiphene is often prescribed along with artificial insemination or assisted reproductive techniques.

How to Use This Drug

The typical starting dose of clomiphene is 50 mg daily for 5 days. Dosing begins on the third, fourth, or fifth day after your period starts. Ovulation may begin 7 days after you have taken the last dose of the drug. If you do not begin to ovulate, the dose can be increased by 50 mg per day each month up to 150 mg or higher, depending on what your doctor prescribes. Once you begin to ovulate, most physicians recommend taking clomiphene for no longer than 6 months. If you have not become pregnant after taking the drug for 6 months, your doctor will likely prescribe a different fertility drug.

Side Effects

- Side effects are typically mild: abdominal fullness, bloating, blurry vision, breast tenderness, dizziness, headache, hot flashes, and nausea.
- Blurry vision or seeing spots or flashes may occur, especially if you are exposed to bright lights. In most cases these vision changes go away within days or weeks of stopping treatment. In rare cases, vision changes are permanent.
- Serious but rare side effects: abnormal vaginal bleeding, mood changes, severe swelling and/or pain in the lower abdomen, sudden and/or rapid weight gain, pain or swelling of the legs, chest pain, and irregular heartbeat.
- Clomiphene may make it more difficult to tell when you are fertile because it can cause changes in the cervical mucus.
- Clomiphene increases the chances of having multiple births.

Possible Drug, Supplement, and/or Food Interactions

No drug, supplement, or food interactions have been found with clomiphene. However, that does not mean interactions cannot occur. If you experience any unusual symptoms while using clomiphene, contact your health-care provider.

Tell Your Doctor

- About any allergies you have, and all prescription and OTC medications you use, as well as supplements.
- If you have ovarian cysts or enlarged ovaries, abnormal vaginal bleeding, liver disease, a pituitary tumor, uncontrolled thyroid or adrenal gland problems, endometriosis, uterine fibroids, or polycystic ovary syndrome.

- If you have been suffering with depression, as clomiphene can make it worse because of hormone changes associated with the drug.

Of Special Interest to Women

- Long-term use of clomiphene citrate may increase the risk of developing ovarian cancer. You should not use clomiphene for more than 6 cycles.
- Approximately 60–80% of women who take clomiphene ovulate, and about 50% get pregnant, usually within 3 cycles.
- This medication is not recommended for women whose ovaries no longer produce eggs properly, typically as a result of ovarian failure or primary pituitary.
- Clomiphene may cause birth defects, so if you think you have become pregnant while taking clomiphene, stop taking the drug and contact your doctor immediately.

Symptoms of Overdose

Abdominal pain, pelvic pain, vision problems, and vomiting.

Clopidogrel

Brand Name

Plavix

Available as Generic?

Yes

Principal Uses

To prevent heart attack and stroke in individuals who have heart disease, recent stroke, or peripheral vascular disease

About the Drug

Clopidogrel is an antiplatelet drug that works by blocking blood cells called platelets from binding together and forming blood clots. It is similar to ticlopidine (Ticlid) both in structure and function. However, unlike ticlopidine, it does not cause significant reductions in white blood cell levels. One large study has shown clopidogrel to be more effective than aspirin in reducing heart attacks. A January 2011 Cochrane Database of Systematic Reviews found clopidogrel plus aspirin to be associated with a reduced risk of cardiovascular events and an increased risk of bleeding compared with aspirin alone.

How to Use This Drug

Clopidogrel is available as tablets. The typical dose is one 75 mg tablet daily, and it can be taken with or without food. Take this medication with a full glass of water. If you have reduced activity of liver enzymes that are necessary to activate clopidogrel, you may not respond adequately to this medication, and your doctor will find an alternative.

Side Effects

- Common side effects: abdominal pain, diarrhea, itching, and rash occur in about 5% of patients. Other common side effects: constipation, dizziness, flulike symptoms, headache, and joint/back pain.
- Unlikely but serious side effects that you should report immediately to your health-care provider: black stools, chest pain, confusion, depression, easy bruising or bleeding, loss of consciousness, persistent stomach pain, persistent nausea or vomiting, slurred speech, unusual weakness, vision changes, vomit that looks like coffee grounds, and yellowing of the skin or eyes.
- In rare cases, clopidogrel causes thrombotic thrombocytopenic purpura (TTP; 1 in 250,000). TTP is characterized by blood clots that develop throughout the body. The related drug ticlopidine causes TTP 17–50 times more frequently than clopidogrel.

Possible Drug, Supplement, and/or Food Interactions

- Daily use of alcohol while taking clopidogrel may increase the risk of stomach bleeding.
- Clopidogrel with NSAIDs, such as diclofenac, ibuprofen, naproxen, and sulindac, may increase the risk of gastrointestinal bleeding.
- The following drugs may reduce the effectiveness of clopidogrel: cimetidine, esomeprazole, felbamate, fluoxetine, fluvoxamine, ketoconazole, omeprazole, and voriconazole.
- High concentrations of clopidogrel in the blood can inhibit the activity of the enzyme that eliminates warfarin, which could result in high levels of warfarin and an increased risk of bleeding.

Tell Your Doctor

- If you have any allergies and all OTC and prescription medications you are taking, as well as supplements.
- If you have a blood disorder (e.g., hemophilia) or bleeding conditions (e.g., active peptic ulcers).
- If you have had recent surgery or a serious physical injury, or if you have severe liver or kidney disease, a history of abnormal bleeding, or other conditions that may put you at increased risk for bleeding (e.g., certain stomach problems).
- If you plan to have surgery, including dental surgery, tell your doctor or dentist that you are taking clopidogrel.

Of Special Interest to Women
- Clopidogrel is in FDA pregnancy Category B, which means it is not expected to harm the fetus. However, it should be used during pregnancy only if your health-care provider decides it is necessary.
- Although studies in rats show that clopidogrel passes into breast milk, it is not known whether it also appears in human breast milk. Breast-feeding while taking clopidogrel is not recommended; consult your health-care provider.

Symptoms of Overdose
Unusual bleeding or bruising.

Clotrimazole

Brand Names
Gyne-Lotrimin, Lotrimin, Mycelex

Available as Generic?
Yes

Principal Uses
Fungal infections caused by *Candida albicans*, for example, vaginal yeast infections and oral thrush

About the Drug
Clotrimazole is an azole antifungal medication that is related to fluconazole (Diflucan), itraconazole (Sporanox), ketoconazole (Nizoral), and miconazole (Micatin, Monistat). Clotrimazole prevents the growth of several types of fungi, especially *Candida albicans,* by stopping the production of the membranes that surround and protect fungal cells. Clotrimazole can be used on the skin, inserted into the vagina, or dissolved in the mouth, depending on the condition for which it is being used.

How to Use This Drug
Clotrimazole is available as a topical cream or lotion (1%), a vaginal suppository, a vaginal cream, and lozenges (called troches). When used on the skin, clotrimazole is typically applied twice daily. The vaginal cream is inserted using an applicator, once daily at night, usually for 7 consecutive days. Two strengths of vaginal suppository are available: The 100 mg dose is inserted once daily, usually at bedtime, for 7 consecutive days; the 200 mg dose is inserted once daily, at bedtime, for 3 days.

If you use the lozenges, allow them to dissolve slowly in your mouth; do not chew them or swallow them whole. The typical treatment course involves taking the lozenges 5 times a day. Clotrimazole lozenges are only for treatment of oral thrush; they do not have an effect on fungal infections anywhere else in your body.

Side Effects

- Common side effects of the creams and lotion: blistering, burning, hives, itching, peeling, redness, stinging, and swelling at the area of application.
- Common side effects of the lozenges: mild itching, nausea, unpleasant sensation in the mouth, and vomiting.

Possible Drug, Supplement, and/or Food Interactions

- Clotrimazole may increase the plasma concentration of fentanyl and result in significant side effects such as confusion, dizziness, extreme sedation, and shortness of breath.
- Clotrimazole may result in high plasma levels of terfenadine, which can lead to ventricular arrhythmias or cardiac arrest.
- Clotrimazole may increase the levels of tacrolimus or sirolimus and result in more serious significant side effects.

Tell Your Doctor

- If you have any allergies, especially to other azole antifungal medications, and also all OTC and prescription medications you are taking, as well as supplements.
- If you have liver disease, HIV or AIDS, diabetes, or a history of alcohol abuse.

Of Special Interest to Women

- Studies of the use of clotrimazole in women during their second and third trimesters have not shown any ill effects, nor have studies of large amounts of intravaginal clotrimazole administered to rats. Consult your health-care provider before using clotrimazole during pregnancy.
- It is not known if clotrimazole passes into breast milk. However, it is known that clotrimazole creams and lotions are very poorly absorbed into the blood and the body when applied to the skin or the vagina.
- While using clotrimazole to treat a vaginal infection, do not engage in sexual intercourse. Also, do not use latex products such as condoms or diaphragms within 72 hours of using this medication because an ingredient in the cream can weaken some latex products.

Symptoms of Overdose

None reported.

Colchicine

Brand Names
None
Available as Generic?
Yes
Principal Uses
Gouty arthritis, for both acute flares and to prevent recurrent acute attacks; also used to treat familial Mediterranean fever, pseudogout, amyloidosis, and scleroderma
About the Drug
Colchicine relieves the inflammation that is characteristic of acute gouty arthritis: Uric acid crystals form in the joints, and this leads to severe pain, swelling, and redness. The joints most often affected are the big toe (majority of cases), as well as the ankle and knee. Colchicine suppresses the inflammation by decreasing the buildup of uric acid crystals.

In people who have familial Mediterranean fever, colchicine is believed to work by decreasing the body's production of a protein called amyloid A that accumulates in people who have this disease. Familial Mediterranean fever is characterized by recurrent fever and painful inflammation of the lungs, abdomen, and joints.
How to Use This Drug
Colchicine is available as tablets and can be taken with or without food. It works best if taken at the first signs of an oncoming attack. For an acute attack, the recommended dose is 1.2 mg at the first sign of an attack, followed by 0.6 mg 1 hour later. You can take additional doses; however, consult your health-care provider ahead of time about how soon you can repeat treatment. If you are taking colchicine to help prevent attacks, 0.6 mg may be taken daily or every 3–4 days, depending on your doctor's recommendations.
Side Effects
- Most common side effects: abdominal pain, diarrhea, nausea, and vomiting.
- Less common side effects: hair loss, nerve irritation, and weakness.
- An infrequent but serious side effect is damage to bone marrow, which can result in severe anemia, low white blood cell counts, and an increased risk of infections. Long-term use of colchicine requires periodic monitoring of blood counts.

Possible Drug, Supplement, and/or Food Interactions
- Erythromycin and clarithromycin may elevate blood levels of colchicine and thus also increase its side effects.
- Do not eat grapefruit or drink grapefruit juice while using colchicine.
- Colchicine can reduce your ability to absorb vitamin B_{12}. Discuss this with your health-care provider.
- Alcohol reduces the effectiveness of colchicine.
- Colchicine rarely causes a serious muscle condition called rhabdomyolysis. Risk of this condition increases if you take other drugs also associated with rhabdomyolysis, including atorvastatin, digoxin, gemfibrozil, fenofibrate, pravastatin, simvastatin.
- Azole antifungals, cyclosporine, HIV medications, macrolide antibiotics, and verapamil with colchicine may increase the risk of serious side effects.

Tell Your Doctor
- If you have any allergies and all prescription and OTC medications you use, as well as supplements.
- If you are pregnant or plan to get pregnant.
- If you have a history of kidney or liver problems.

Of Special Interest to Women
- Colchicine can stop cell division, so it should not be used during pregnancy because it may affect fetal growth. However, no adequate studies have been done in pregnant women.
- Colchicine passes into breast milk. Although there have not been any reports of harmful effects to nursing infants, consult your health-care provider before using this drug while breast-feeding. He or she may recommend that you allow a specific amount of time between when you take your medication and when you breast-feed.
- Colchicine may interfere with the results of certain lab tests, possibly giving you false results. Tell all your doctors and lab personnel that you are using this drug before you undergo lab tests.

Symptoms of Overdose
Abdominal pain, breathing difficulties, severe diarrhea, severe nausea, weakness, severe vomiting.

Conjugated Estrogens

Brand Names

Cenestin, Enjuvia, Premarin

Available as Generic?

No

Principal Uses

Menopausal symptoms, whether due to natural menopause or removal of the ovaries, ovarian failure, or underdevelopment of organs that secrete hormones (hypogonadism)

About the Drug

Conjugated estrogens are a mixture of several different estrogens derived from the urine of pregnant mares. The main components are sodium estrone sulphate and sodium equilin sulfate.

How to Use This Drug

Conjugated estrogens are available as tablets and vaginal cream. Intravenous or intramuscular injections are reserved for treatment of abnormal uterine bleeding due to hormonal imbalance and must be given by a health-care professional.

To minimize side effects, your health-care provider should prescribe the lowest possible oral dose. The usual starting dose for treating menopausal symptoms is 0.3 mg/day. Your doctor may prescribe them on a continuous basis or cyclical intervals (e.g., 25 days of treatment, then 5 days off).

For hypogonadism, typical dosing is 0.3 mg or 0.625 mg daily following a schedule of 25 days of treatment and then 5 days off. Women who have ovarian failure are usually prescribed 1.25 mg daily for 3 weeks followed by 1 week off. However, because symptoms often return during the week off, many women take conjugated estrogens continuously.

The vaginal cream can be used to treat vulvar and vaginal atrophy at a suggested dose of ½–2 g daily.

Side Effects

In addition to the following side effects, see "Of Special Interest to Women" below, regarding the findings of the Women's Health Initiative and complications associated with estrogen therapy.

- Common side effects: abdominal pain, back pain, breast pain, breast enlargement, brown patches on the skin, decreased sex drive, headache, heartburn, loss of periods or excessively prolonged periods, joint pain, nausea, nervousness, rash, and vaginal bleeding or spotting.

- Less common side effects: depression, diarrhea, dizziness, gas, insomnia, leg cramps, sinusitis, and vaginitis.
- Conjugated estrogens can increase the curvature of the cornea, so if you wear contact lenses, you may develop an inability to wear them.
- Use of conjugated estrogens also carries a risk of salt and water retention, an increase in blood pressure and triglyceride levels, yellowing of the skin or eyes, and an increased risk of cholesterol gallstones.

Possible Drug, Supplement, and/or Food Interactions

- Conjugated estrogens increase the liver's ability to make substances that promote blood clotting. Therefore, if you are taking a blood thinner (e.g., warfarin), you should be monitored for reduced ability of warfarin to thin your blood.
- The following drugs increase the elimination of estrogen from the body and thus may reduce its beneficial effects: barbiturates, carbamazepine, griseofulvin, phenytoin, primidone, rifampin, and Saint-John's-wort.
- Erythromycin, itraconazole, ketoconazole, and ritonavir may increase the levels of estrogens in the blood.
- Avoid grapefruit juice and grapefruit, which may increase estrogen levels in the blood and result in more side effects.

Tell Your Doctor

- If you have any allergies and all prescription or OTC medications you are taking, as well as supplements.
- If you have a history of heart attack, stroke, or blood clots; abnormal vaginal bleeding that has not been checked by a physician; liver disease; or any type of breast, uterine, or hormone-dependent cancer. You should not take conjugated estrogens if you have any of these conditions.
- If you have asthma, circulation problems, diabetes, epilepsy or other seizure disorder, endometriosis, gallbladder disease, heart disease, high blood pressure, high cholesterol or triglycerides, high or low calcium levels, kidney disease, lupus, migraines, porphyria, or underactive thyroid (hypothyroidism), or if you have had a hysterectomy.
- If you are a vegetarian. You may want to ask for an alternative estrogen that does not contain animal ingredients.

Of Special Interest to Women

- Conjugated estrogens are an FDA pregnancy Category X medication, because they are known to cause birth defects. Tell your doctor immediately if you become pregnant while taking this medication.
- Use an effective form of birth control while using conjugated estrogens.
- Estrogens are secreted in breast milk and can cause unpredictable effects in infants. Do not take conjugated estrogens if you are breast-feeding.
- The Women's Health Initiative found that postmenopausal women ages 50–79 who took conjugated estrogens (0.625 mg/day) along with medroxyprogesterone (2.5 mg/day) for 5 years had an increased risk of heart attack, stroke, blood clots, and breast cancer. Women who took conjugated estrogens without progesterone experienced an increased risk of stroke only. Women older than 65 also had an increased risk of impaired cognition and/or dementia when taking estrogens alone or estrogens and medroxyprogesterone. However, you should also note that aside from the WHI, conjugated estrogens are associated with an increased risk of blood clots in the legs and endometrial cancer. Long-term use of conjugated estrogens may also increase your risk of stroke, especially if you are overweight or smoke. You should be checked regularly (every 3–6 months) if you are on prolonged estrogen treatment and you have risk factors for stroke and blood clots.
- If you take conjugated estrogens and smoke, you have a higher risk of life-threatening blood clots.

Symptoms of Overdose

Nausea, vaginal bleeding, and vomiting.

Cyclobenzaprine

Brand Names

Flexeril, Amrix

Available as Generic?

Yes

Principal Uses

Short-term relief of muscle spasms associated with acute painful muscle and skeletal conditions, such as fibromyalgia

About the Drug

Cyclobenzaprine is a muscle relaxant that relieves muscle spasm that is related to the muscle itself and not to the nerves that control the muscles. The medication appears to work through a complex relationship with the nervous system, likely the brain stem. Cyclobenzaprine works best when combined with rest and physical therapy. Research shows it can significantly reduce pain and muscle tightness associated with fibromyalgia.

How to Use This Drug

Cyclobenzaprine is available as tablets and extended-release capsules. The typical dose is 5–10 mg 3 times daily of the immediate-release tablets, or 15–30 mg once daily of the extended-release capsules. This medication is intended for use no longer than 3 weeks unless your doctor gives you other instructions.

Side Effects

- Common side effects: dizziness, drowsiness, dry mouth, fatigue, headache, and light-headedness.
- Less common side effects: abdominal pain, acid reflux, blurry vision, confusion, constipation, nausea, nervousness, and unpleasant taste.
- If you abruptly stop taking cyclobenzaprine after long-term use, you may experience headache, nausea, and weakness.
- Contact your health-care provider immediately if you experience abdominal pain, dark urine, difficulty urinating, fainting, fast or irregular heartbeat, mental/mood changes such as confusion or hallucinations, persistent nausea/vomiting, seizures, or yellowing of the skin or eyes.

Possible Drug, Supplement, and/or Food Interactions

- Cyclobenzaprine may interact with antianxiety drugs (e.g., diazepam), antihistamines that cause drowsiness (e.g., diphenhydramine), antiseizure drugs (e.g., carbamazepine) sedatives, narcotic pain relievers, and psychiatric medications (e.g., phenothiazines).
- Cyclobenzaprine may interact with substances and medications that slow the brain's processes, such as alcohol, barbiturates, and benzodiazepines.
- Do not take cyclobenzaprine with or within 2 weeks of any MAOIs, such as isocarboxazid, phenelzine, procarbazine, or tranylcypromine. This interaction can result in high fever, convulsions, and death.

Tell Your Doctor

- If you have any allergies and all OTC and prescription medications you are taking, as well as supplements.

- If you are taking asthma drugs (e.g., albuterol, salmeterol), cimetidine, clonidine, guanethidine, guanadrel, SSRI antidepressants (e.g., citalopram, fluoxetine), stimulants and diet pills (e.g., ephedrine, phenylephrine) tramadol, tricyclic antidepressants (e.g., amitriptyline, imipramine).
- If you have hyperthyroidism, irregular heartbeat or other heart problems, a recent heart attack, or moderate or severe liver disease you should not take cyclobenzaprine.
- If you have severe difficulty urinating, glaucoma, or mild liver disease.

Of Special Interest to Women
- Although no adequate studies have been done in pregnant women, animal studies have not shown any important effects of cyclobenzaprine on the fetus. Therefore, you and your health-care provider can discuss the possibility of taking the drug while you are pregnant.
- It is not known whether cyclobenzaprine is secreted in milk. However, because it is related to tricyclic antidepressants, which can be passed in breast milk, discuss this question with your health-care provider.

Symptoms of Overdose
Chest pain, fast heartbeat, hallucinations, increased muscle stiffness with fever and sweating, severe drowsiness, and slurred speech.

Cyclophosphamide

Brand Name
Cytoxan

Available as Generic?
Yes

Principal Uses
Several types of cancer, often in combination with other drugs for breast cancer, ovarian cancer, and leukemia; various off-label uses of interest to women (see "About the Drug")

About the Drug
Cyclophosphamide is a chemotherapy drug and an immunosuppressive drug used primarily for treating various types of cancer. Once cyclophosphamide is ingested, the liver converts it into two chemicals, acrolein and phosphoramide, which slow the growth of cancer by disrupting the DNA within cancer cells. Because cyclophosphamide can destroy

cancer cells, it is referred to as a cytotoxic drug; unfortunately, this drug also destroys normal cells, resulting in often serious side effects.

Cyclophosphamide also reduces your immune system's response to various diseases. Therefore, in addition to treatment of cancer, cyclophosphamide is often prescribed for off-label uses, including treatment of advanced mycosis fungoides, lupus, rheumatoid arthritis, vasculitis, and Wegener's granulomatosis.

How to Use This Drug

Cyclophosphamide is available in tablets and as a powder for intravenous injection. The typical initial dose for adults is 40–50 mg/kg given intravenously over 3–5 days in divided doses. The usual oral dose is 1–5 mg/kg daily. Your doctor will adjust your subsequent maintenance doses based on how you respond to treatment.

While taking cyclophosphamide, you should drink more fluids than you normally do to help avoid kidney and bladder side effects. It is best to take the tablets on an empty stomach if possible. If you experience stomach upset, take the tablets with food. The best times to take cyclophosphamide are in the morning or afternoon, as taking them at night may increase your risk of bladder damage.

Side Effects

- Common side effects: diarrhea, hair loss, mouth sores, sterility, vomiting, and yellowing of the skin or eyes.
- Unlikely side effects: bloody urine, cessation of menstrual periods, easy bruising or bleeding, joint pain, and unusual tiredness or weakness.
- Rare but serious side effects that should be reported to your healthcare provider: bloody stools, breathing difficulties, chest pain, dark urine, painful urination, irregular heartbeat, mental/mood changes, muscle weakness or spasm, night sweats, pelvic pain, severe abdominal pain, signs of infection (e.g., fever, chills), swelling of the ankles, swollen glands, unusual growths or lumps, and yellowing of the eyes or skin.
- Cyclophosphamide can cause kidney failure and may also damage the heart and lungs. It can cause inflammation of the urinary bladder with bleeding, resulting in lower-abdominal pain, anemia, and problems with urination.
- Cyclophosphamide suppresses blood cell production and may cause anemia, thrombocytopenia (reduced platelets), and leukopenia (reduced white blood cells). It also reduces the body's ability to fight infections.

- Some patients are at increased risk of developing another form of cancer (besides the one they are being treated for) months to years after treatment. Talk to your doctor about this potential side effect.

Possible Drug, Supplement, and/or Food Interactions

- Cyclophosphamide with nalidixic acid may cause very serious interactions.
- The following medications and herbal remedies may interact with cyclophosphamide: chloramphenicol, chloroquine, digoxin, phenobarbital, phenothiazines, Saint-John's-wort, and turmeric.
- Allopurinol (Zyloprim) increases the ability of cyclophosphamide to reduce production of blood cells.
- Cyclophosphamide increases the action of blood thinners such as warfarin and decreases the effects of quinolone antibiotics (e.g., ciprofloxacin).

Tell Your Doctor

- If you have any allergies and all OTC and prescription medications you are taking, as well as supplements.
- If you have decreased bone marrow function (e.g., anemia, leukopenia), liver disease, or kidney disease.
- Before you get any immunizations or vaccinations, and avoid contact with anyone who has recently received oral polio vaccine.

Of Special Interest to Women

- This drug is not recommended during pregnancy as fetuses exposed to cyclophosphamide may be born with missing fingers, toes, and/or a poorly developed heart.
- If you are of childbearing age, use reliable birth control during treatment with cyclophosphamide.
- Cyclophosphamide passes into breast milk and may cause harm to a nursing infant. Consult your doctor before breast-feeding.
- Because cyclophosphamide can be absorbed through the skin, do not handle or break these tablets if you are pregnant.
- Sterility is usually temporary with cyclophosphamide, but in some women it can be permanent. Consult your health-care provider for more details.

Symptoms of Overdose

Increased susceptibility to infections and heart damage.

Cyclosporine Ophthalmic Emulsion

Brand Name
Restasis

Available as Generic?
No

Principal Uses
Chronic dry eye; also associated with Sjögren's syndrome

About the Drug
Cyclosporine ophthalmic emulsion helps increase your eyes' natural ability to produce tears, which may be hampered by inflammation associated with chronic dry eye. It does not increase the production of tears if you are using anti-inflammatory eyedrops or tear duct plugs. The drug has not been studied in people who have a history of herpes viral infections of the eye.

How to Use This Drug
Cyclosporine ophthalmic emulsion is available in single-use vials. To administer the drops:

1. Wash your hands thoroughly with soap and water.
2. Turn the vial over several times until the liquid inside looks white.
3. Open the vial—avoid touching the dropper against your eye or any other surface.
4. Using the index finger of one hand, pull the lower lid of your eye down to form a pocket. Drop the number of drops prescribed by your doctor into the pocket. Placing the drops on your eyeball can cause stinging.
5. Close your eye and press lightly against your lower lid with your finger for 2–3 minutes.
6. Discard any unused medication in the vial.

These eyedrops are typically prescribed for use twice daily. Do not use cyclosporine ophthalmic emulsion if you have an active eye infection or when you are wearing contact lenses. If you are a contact lens wearer, wait at least 15 minutes after administering the eyedrops before you insert your contacts.

Side Effects
- Common side effect: temporary burning sensation in the eye(s), which affects about 17% of patients.
- Other side effects: blurry vision, discharge, eye pain, eye redness, foreign body sensation in the eye, itching, stinging, and watery eyes.

Possible Drug, Supplement, and/or Food Interactions
- Do not use cyclosporine ophthalmic emulsion if you are also using other eyedrops or medications without consulting your physician.
- If you are using other eyedrops specifically for dry eyes (e.g., artificial tears), wait at least 15 minutes between use of the two products.

Tell Your Doctor
- If you have any allergies, especially to cyclosporine.
- About all prescription and OTC medications you use, as well as supplements.
- If you have an eye infection, a punctal plug, or have ever had a herpes eye infection.

Of Special Interest to Women
- This medication should be used during pregnancy only if you and your doctor decide the benefits outweigh the risks.
- It is not known whether cyclosporine ophthalmic emulsion passes into breast milk. Discuss breast-feeding with your health-care provider.

Symptoms of Overdose
An overdose is unlikely. If you believe you have administered too much of the medication, wash your eye out with water and contact your physician.

Denosumab

Brand Name
Prolia

Available as Generic?
No

Principal Use
Osteoporosis in postmenopausal women who have an increased risk for fractures and who cannot use other osteoporosis medications or for whom other osteoporosis medications have not been effective

About the Drug
Denosumab is a monoclonal antibody. It works by slowing bone loss to help maintain bone strength and to reduce the risk of fractures. Specifically, denosumab prevents cells called osteoclasts from breaking down bone.

How to Use This Drug
Denosumab is injected under the skin of the upper arm, abdomen, or upper thigh by a physician or nurse every 6 months. The injection can

be given at a doctor's office, hospital, or clinic. Use of denosumab should be accompanied by daily supplementation with vitamin D (usually 400 IU) and calcium (usually 1000 mg).

Side Effects

- Common side effects: back pain, bladder infection, high cholesterol, muscle pain, and pain in the arms and legs.
- Less common side effects: skin reactions such as dryness, peeling, itching, rash, eczema, or dermatitis (inflammation of the skin). Because these reactions may also be signs of severe allergic reactions, seek medical help immediately if you develop a rash or if any of these symptoms persist or get worse.
- Serious side effects: hypocalcemia (low calcium levels in the blood); endocarditis (inflammation of the inner lining of the heart); and serious infections of the skin, ear, abdomen, or bladder.
- Severe jawbone problems (osteonecrosis) may occur. Some studies indicate that about 2% of postmenopausal women and/or women with breast cancer using denosumab have developed osteonecrosis.

Possible Drug, Supplement, and/or Food Interactions

No specific interactions have been documented at this time. Tell your doctor about any medications or supplements you are taking before you are treated with denosumab.

Tell Your Doctor

- If you have any allergies and all OTC and/or prescription medications you are taking, as well as supplements.
- If you have low blood calcium, kidney problems, multiple myeloma, or difficulty absorbing minerals in your stomach or intestinal tract (malabsorption syndrome). Also tell your doctor if you have had parathyroid or thyroid surgery, if you are on kidney dialysis, or if you are unable to take daily calcium and vitamin D.
- If you plan to have dental surgery or tooth extraction, tell your doctor and dentist before you take denosumab. Poor dental hygiene, poorly fitting dentures, gum disease, and anemia can increase your risk of osteonecrosis.

Of Special Interest to Women

- Denosumab should not be used during pregnancy, as it may harm the fetus.
- It is not known if denosumab passes into breast milk. Consult your doctor before breast-feeding.

- Undergo periodic lab and/or medical tests (e.g., bone density; calcium, phosphorus, and magnesium levels; kidney function) while you are using denosumab.

Symptoms of Overdose

An overdose is highly unlikely, because it is administered by a medical professional using a single-dose, prefilled vial or syringe.

Diazepam

Brand Names

Valium, Diastat

Available as Generic?

Yes

Principal Uses

Anxiety, panic disorders, seizures, and acute alcohol withdrawal

About the Drug

Diazepam is a benzodiazepine, one of the top two most frequently abused group of prescription drugs in the United States (opioids are the other), according to the Drug Abuse Warning Network, which monitors medications and illicit drugs that are reported to emergency departments. Benzodiazepines are also among the prescription drugs most abused by women. Other benzodiazepines include alprazolam (Xanax), clonazepam (Klonopin), flurazepam (Dalmane), lorazepam (Ativan), and temazepan (Restoril).

Diazepam affects the brain and central nervous system by boosting the influence of the brain chemical GABA (gamma-aminobutyric acid), which inhibits activity in the brain. Experts believe that excessive brain activity may lead to anxiety.

How to Use This Drug

Diazepam is available as tablets, liquid, rectal gel, and via injection. The oral doses may be taken with or without food. The usual oral dose is 2–10 mg taken 2–4 times daily. The usual rectal dose is 0.2–0.5 mg/kg and depends on your age.

If you take the liquid form, use the medication measuring device provided; never use a household spoon because you will not get the proper dose. The liquid medication can be added to liquid or soft food immediately before taking it.

Diazepam can be habit-forming. If you suddenly stop taking diazepam, you may experience withdrawal symptoms, including muscle cramps, sleep problems, stomach pain, sweating, tremor, unusual thoughts or behaviors, and vomiting. Consult your doctor to establish a tapering-off program.

Side Effects

- Common side effects: blurry vision, constipation, dizziness, drowsiness, fatigue, headache, and trouble breathing.
- Less likely but serious side effects: decreased interest in sex, clumsiness, mental/mood changes (e.g., agitation, hallucinations, memory problems), sleep problems, slurred speech, tremors, trouble urinating, and trouble walking.
- Contact your doctor immediately if you experience abdominal pain, dark urine, persistent nausea, persistent sore throat or fever, vomiting, yellowing of the skin or eyes.

Possible Drug, Supplement, and/or Food Interactions

- Drinking alcohol while taking diazepam can make you very drowsy.
- Sodium oxybate or fluvoxamine with diazepam can lead to very serious side effects.
- Diazepam can affect the results of certain lab tests. Tell your health-care provider and lab personnel that you are using this drug.
- Smoking can reduce the effectiveness of diazepam. Your health-care provider may need to adjust your dose.
- Diazepam may react with the herb kava.
- Certain antidepressants (e.g., fluoxetin, nefazodone), cimetidine, clozapine, digoxin, disulfiram, ketoconazole, levodopa, omeprazole, and phenytoin can prolong the effects of diazepam.
- Drugs that cause drowsiness may make this side effect worse. These drugs include antihistamines (e.g., diphenhydramine), antiseizure drugs (e.g., carbamazepine), sedatives, muscle relaxants, narcotic pain relievers, psychiatric medications (e.g., phenothiazines), and tranquilizers.
- Do not eat grapefruit or drink grapefruit juice while using diazepam, as they may increase the amount of the drug in your system.

Tell Your Doctor

- If you have any allergies, especially to other benzodiazepines.
- About all prescription and OTC medications you take, as well as supplements.
- If you have glaucoma (narrow angle), myasthenia gravis, or sleep apnea. Diazepam should not be used if you have these conditions.
- If you have a history of liver disease, kidney disease, lung or breathing problems, drug or alcohol abuse, or glaucoma (open angle).

Of Special Interest to Women
- Diazepam is not recommended during pregnancy because it may harm the fetus. If you are pregnant or become pregnant while taking diazepam, inform your doctor immediately.
- Diazepam passes into breast milk and may cause adverse effects on a nursing infant. Talk to your doctor before breast-feeding.

Symptoms of Overdose

Fainting, loss of consciousness, slowed breathing, slowed reflexes, and severe drowsiness.

Digoxin

Brand Names

Cardoxin, Digitek, Lanoxicaps, Lanoxin

Available as Generic?

Yes

Principal Uses

Mild to moderate congestive heart failure, abnormal heart rhythm (atrial fibrillation)

About the Drug

Digoxin is derived from the leaves of the digitalis plant and belongs to the drug class cardiac glycosides. It is usually used with other medications to make the heart beat stronger and in regular rhythm. Digoxin inhibits the activity of the enzyme ATPase, which controls the movement of specific minerals (e.g., calcium, sodium, potassium) into heart muscle, which in turn reduces stress on the heart and helps it maintain a normal heartbeat.

Digoxin also has the ability to slow down electrical conduction between the chambers of the heart (atria and ventricles), which makes it useful in treating abnormally rapid atrial rhythms such as atrial fibrillation, atrial tachycardia, and atrial flutter.

How to Use This Drug

Digoxin is available in tablets and liquid. If you take the liquid form, use the measuring device provided with the prescription; do not use a household spoon because you will not get the correct dose. The typical starting dose is 0.0625–0.25 mg daily, depending on your age and kidney function. Because digoxin is mainly eliminated by the kidneys, your health-care provider may reduce your dose if you have kidney problems.

It is best to take digoxin at least 2 hours before or after eating certain foods or taking specific medications (see "Possible Drug, Supplement, and/or Food Interactions" below). Do not suddenly stop taking digoxin without talking to your doctor, as some conditions may become worse.

Side Effects

- Common side effects: diarrhea, dizziness, headache, mental changes, nausea, rash, and vomiting.
- Less common side effects: abdominal pain and visual disturbances.
- Serious side effects: heart block, rapid heartbeat, and slow heart rate.
- Although digoxin is used to treat a specific type of abnormal heartbeat, it can cause other types of irregular heartbeat. Contact your health-care provider immediately if you experience unusually fast, slow, or irregular heartbeat.

Possible Drug, Supplement, and/or Food Interactions

- Take digoxin at least 2 hours before or after eating foods that are high in fiber or if you are taking cholestyramine, colestipol, or psyllium.
- If you are taking antacids, kaolin-pectin, milk of magnesia, metoclopramide, sulfasalazine, or aminosalicylic acid, take them as far apart from your dose of digoxin as possible. Consult your pharmacist or physician if you are not sure when to take these medications.
- Diuretics can affect the balance of certain minerals in the body and also how digoxin works, and also result in abnormal heart rhythms.
- Drugs that can increase digoxin levels and the risk of toxicity include alprazolam, amiodarone, indomethacin, itraconazole, quinidine, ritonavir, saquinavir, spironolactone, and verapamil.
- Digoxin with beta-blockers (e.g., propranol) or calcium channel blockers (e.g., verapamil) can cause serious slowing of the heart rate.

Tell Your Doctor

- If you have a history of heart attack, certain heart conditions (e.g., AV block), kidney problems, thyroid problems, or mineral imbalance. The balance of calcium, magnesium, and potassium can affect how digoxin works.
- If you have recently experienced diarrhea or vomiting.
- Before undergoing surgery or certain heart procedures (e.g., electrical cardioversion), or dental surgery, tell your doctor or dentist that you are taking digoxin.

Of Special Interest to Women

- No adequate studies of digoxin in pregnant women have been done. Discuss the benefits and risks of using digoxin with your health-care provider if you are pregnant or plan to get pregnant.

- Digoxin is secreted in breast milk. Discuss the benefits and risks associated with the use of digoxin with your health-care provider if you are breast-feeding or plan to do so.

Symptoms of Overdose

Abnormal heartbeat (very fast, very slow, irregular); dizziness; fainting; and severe diarrhea, nausea, and/or vomiting.

Donepezil

Brand Name

Aricept

Available as Generic?

No

Principal Use

Mild to moderate dementia related to Alzheimer's disease

About the Drug

Donepezil is a cholinesterase inhibitor. This drug is prescribed for dementia associated with Alzheimer's disease because some experts believe this condition may be caused by a deficiency of neurotransmitters, chemicals that allow nerves in the brain to communicate with each other. Donepezil inhibits the enzyme acetylcholinesterase, which is involved in the destruction of the neurotransmitter acetylcholine. Donepezil can increase concentrations of acetylcholine, which in turn may help patients who have dementia. Although donepezil may improve symptoms (memory, the ability to perform daily functions, awareness), it cannot cure Alzheimer's disease.

Based on estimates from the Aging, Demographics, and Memory Study (2007), 14% of all people age 71 and older have dementia, and women have a higher rate than men: 16% versus 11%, respectively. In 2007, researchers using data from the original Framingham Heart Study also looked at the risk of dementia and found that more than 20% of women reaching age 65 eventually developed dementia, compared with 17% of men.

How to Use This Drug

Donepezil is available as traditional and orally disintegrating tablets. The medication is typically taken once a day just prior to going to bed. You can take it with or without food. If you experience insomnia related to donepezil, your doctor may switch you to a morning dose. It typically takes several weeks before the full benefits of donepezil take effect.

Side Effects

- Common side effects: diarrhea, dizziness, fatigue, general pain, headache, increased frequency of urination, insomnia, joint pain, loss of appetite, nausea, and vomiting. These effects typically disappear 1–3 weeks after starting treatment. If they persist or get worse, contact your physician.
- Less likely but serious side effects that should be reported to your physician immediately: black stools, fainting, increased urination, irregular/slow heartbeat, mental/mood changes, seizures, severe stomach pain, vomit that looks like coffee grounds, and weight loss.

Possible Drug, Supplement, and/or Food Interactions

- Anticholinergic medications that can cross into the brain, such as atropine, benztropine, and trihexyphenidyl, counteract the effects of donepezil.
- Medications that reduce the effects of donepezil because they increase the elimination of the drug from the body include carbamazepine, dexamethasone, phenobarbital, phenytoin, and rifampin.
- Ketoconazole and quinidine can increase concentrations of donepezil and cause side effects.
- NSAIDs with donepezil can increase your risk for gastrointestinal bleeding.
- Donepezil with bupropion, iodinated contrast media, sodium phosphate/sodium biphosphates (e.g., enemas such as Fleet Enema), and tramadol may cause seizures.

Tell Your Doctor

- If you have any allergies and all OTC and prescription medications you are taking, as well as supplements.
- If you have breathing problems, gastrointestinal disorders, heart disease, or seizures.

Of Special Interest to Women

- Donepezil is typically prescribed for older women who are past childbearing age. However, if pregnancy is a possibility, discuss the benefits and risks of taking donepezil with your health-care provider. It is not known whether donepezil can harm the fetus.
- It is not known whether donepezil passes into breast milk.

Symptoms of Overdose

Excessive sweating, slow or shallow breathing, seizures, severe or persistent nausea/vomiting, and very slow heartbeat.

Drospirenone/Ethinyl Estradiol

Brand Names

Yasmin 28, Beyaz

Available as Generic?

No

Principal Uses

Prevent pregnancy, treat symptoms of premenstrual dysphoric disorder for women who use an oral contraceptive, and treatment of moderate acne for women who use an oral contraceptive

About the Drug

Drospirenone/ethinyl estradiol is an oral contraceptive regimen that contains the hormones estrogen and progestin. The dosing program consists of 24 tablets that contain 3 mg of drospirenone and 0.02 mg of ethinyl estradiol, plus 4 inert tablets. The active tablets suppress gonadotropins, which inhibit ovulation and change the cervical mucus and endometrium, making it more difficult for sperm to both enter the uterus and to implant in the uterine wall. These tablets can also help make your periods more regular, reduce cramping during your period, and decrease your risk of ovarian cysts.

A second type of drospirenone/ethinyl estradiol regimen also contains levomefolate calcium, a folate supplement (Beyaz). This product is for women who want to use an oral contraceptive that increases their folate levels for the purpose of reducing their risk of neural tube birth defects. In addition to the drospirenone and ethinyl estradiol, these tablets contain 0.451 mg levomefolate calcium in both the active and inert tablets.

How to Use This Drug

Drospirenone/ethinyl estradiol is available as tablets and should be taken once daily and at the same time each day. You increase your risk of pregnancy if you miss a pill or if you take your pills at different times of the day. You can take the medication with food if it bothers your stomach.

Begin taking the pills on the day your health-care provider recommends. When you first begin taking this medication, use an additional form of nonhormonal birth control for the first 7 days until the medication has a chance to work. Take 1 pill each day, including the inert tablets. You should get your period during the fourth week of the cycle. If you do not, consult your doctor.

Side Effects
- Common side effects: bloating, breast tenderness or enlargement, dizziness, headache, increased vaginal fluids, nausea, stomach cramps, vaginal bleeding between periods (spotting), vaginal discomfort, and vomiting.
- If you have acne, it may improve or get worse when taking this medication.
- Unlikely but serious side effects that you should report immediately to your doctor: changes in vaginal bleeding (e.g., sudden heavy bleeding, missed periods), dark patches on your skin, discomfort wearing contact lenses, swelling of the ankles or feet, unwanted facial and/or body hair, and weight changes.
- Rare but very serious side effects that should be reported immediately to your doctor: chest pain, confusion, coughing up blood, dark urine, headaches that differ from those you have had in the past, jaw and/or left arm pain, lumps in your breast, mental/mood changes, numbness in the arms or legs, pain/swelling/warmth in the groin or calf, slurred speech, sudden dizziness/fainting, sudden shortness of breath, unusual tiredness, vision changes, weakness on one side of the body, or yellowing of the eyes or skin.

Possible Drug, Supplement, and/or Food Interactions
- The following medications with drospirenone/ethinyl estradiol may cause very serious interactions: aromatase inhibitors (e.g., anastrazole), sodium tetradecyl sulfate, and troleandomycin.
- Drugs that may decrease the effectiveness of drospirenone/ethinyl estradiol include many antibiotics (e.g., cephalosporins, erythromycin, penicillins, sulfas), aprepitant, bexarotene, dapsone, griseofulvin, some HIV protease inhibitors (e.g., amprenavir, ritonavir), nevirapine, rifamycins, many seizure medications (e.g., barbiturates, phenytoin), and the herb Saint-John's-wort.
- Drospirenone/ethinyl estradiol may slow or accelerate the elimination of other drugs from your body. Those drugs include acetaminophen, aspirin, some beta-blockers (e.g., metoprolol), cyclosporine, morphine, corticosteroids such as prednisolone, some benzodiazepines (e.g., lorazepam), and theophylline.
- Drugs that can increase the blood levels of drospirenone/ethinyl estradiol include acetaminophen, atorvastatin, azole antifungals (e.g., itraconazole), and vitamin C.

Tell Your Doctor

- If you have any allergies, especially to ethinyl estradiol, drospirenone, other estrogens or progestins, or spironolactone.
- All OTC and prescription medications you are taking.
- If you smoke. If you are older than 35 and smoke, you should not use this birth control method.
- Before undergoing lab tests, tell your doctor and lab personnel that you are taking drospirenone/ethinyl estradiol, because it can affect your test results.
- If you have high cholesterol or triglyceride levels, depression, swelling, gallbladder problems, migraines, obesity, irregular/missed/very light periods, recent pregnancy, or thyroid problems.
- If you have any of the following conditions, because you should not use this method of birth control: history of stroke or blood clots, high blood pressure, abnormal breast exam, cancer, diabetes, severe headaches, history of heart disease, kidney problems, liver problems, are pregnant, recent major surgery, immobility, history of yellowing of the eyes or skin while pregnant or while using birth control pills, unexplained vaginal bleeding, or heavy tobacco use.
- If you are scheduled for surgery. Your doctor may want you to stop taking drospirenone for a while.

Of Special Interest to Women

- If you become pregnant while taking this medication or suspect you may be pregnant, contact your health-care provider immediately.
- This medication passes into breast milk and may harm a nursing infant. You should not breast-feed.
- If you miss two periods in a row while taking this medication, contact your doctor for a pregnancy test.
- It may take longer to become pregnant after you stop taking this medication.

Symptoms of Overdose

Severe nausea and vomiting and sudden or unusual vaginal bleeding.

Duloxetine

Brand Name

Cymbalta

Available as Generic?

No

Principal Uses

Anxiety disorder, major depression, fibromyalgia, diabetic peripheral neuropathy

About the Drug

Duloxetine is an SNRI and one of the few drugs approved by the FDA for fibromyalgia. Other drugs in this class include desvenlafaxine (Pristiq), milnacipran (Savella; also approved for fibromyalgia), and venlafaxine (Effexor).

Duloxetine acts on the neurotransmitters serotonin and epinephrine, chemicals in the brain that facilitate communication between nerves. An imbalance among neurotransmitters is believed to be a cause of depression and other psychiatric disorders. Duloxetine prevents the reuptake of serotonin and norepinephrine by nerves after these chemicals have been released by nerves in the brain. This increases the impact serotonin and norepinephrine have on the brain, which improves mood.

Exactly why duloxetine is effective in treating pain caused by fibromyalgia is not known, but experts believe it is associated with the drug's impact on serotonin and norepinephrine in the brain.

How to Use This Drug

Duloxetine is available in capsules, which should be swallowed whole and never chewed or crushed. The recommended dose for depression is 20 mg or 30 mg twice daily or 60 mg once a day. Patients often begin at a low dose, which can be increased as needed to 60 mg daily. Although you can take this medication with or without food, taking it with food may reduce feelings of nausea, which can occur when starting treatment. For anxiety disorder or pain associated with fibromyalgia or diabetic neuropathy, the typical dose is 60 mg daily. Higher doses do not appear to provide any additional benefit. Always take duloxetine at the same time each day. It can take up to 4 weeks to feel the full effects of duloxetine.

Duloxetine can cause withdrawal symptoms if you stop taking it suddenly. Consult your doctor before stopping this medication to help you reduce your dose gradually.

Side Effects

- Common side effects: blurry vision, constipation, diarrhea, difficulty sleeping, dizziness, dry mouth, fatigue, nausea, and yawning.
- Unlikely but serious side effects may occur; contact your doctor immediately: elevated blood pressure, fainting, decreased sex drive, difficulty urinating or a change in the amount of urine, thoughts of suicide, tremors, unusual or severe mental/mood changes, and weight loss.

- Rare but very serious side effects that require immediate medical attention: stomach pain, bloody and/or tarry stools, vomit that looks like coffee grounds, easy bleeding and/or bruising, yellowing of the eyes and/or skin, dark urine, seizures, and irregular heartbeat.
- Some people experience withdrawal symptoms when they stop taking duloxetine. These can include anxiety, insomnia, nausea, and nervousness. Withdrawal from duloxetine should be done gradually to help prevent these symptoms.
- Serotonin syndrome may be more likely to occur when you start or increase the dose of duloxetine. Symptoms include hallucinations, rapid heartbeat, severe dizziness, unexplained fever, severe nausea/vomiting, severe diarrhea, loss of coordination, and restlessness. Seek immediate medical help.

Possible Drug, Supplement, and/or Food Interactions

- Duloxetine with MAOIs such as phenelzine (Nardil), selegiline (Eldepryl), or tranylcypromine (Parnate), or within 14 days of stopping MAOIs, can be fatal.
- Duloxetine with antipsychotics, tricyclic antidepressants, or other drugs that have an effect on serotonin in the brain, such as tryptophan and sumatriptan (Imitrex), may cause serotonin syndrome, which is characterized by hallucinations, very high body temperature, extreme agitation, muscle rigidity, coma, and even death.
- Duloxetine should not be taken with Saint-John's-wort, because this herb can affect serotonin levels.
- Fluoxetine (Prozac), paroxetine (Paxil), fluvoxamine (Luvox), and quinidine (Quinidine) can increase the blood levels of duloxetine, which may increase the risk of side effects.
- Avoid taking duloxetine with aspirin, NSAIDs, warfarin (Coumadin), and other drugs that are associated with bleeding.
- Duloxetine can cause drowsiness; therefore, taking other drugs that are associated with drowsiness can increase the effect. These include certain antihistamines (e.g., diphenhydramine), antiseizure drugs (e.g., carbamazepine), medications for sleep or anxiety (e.g., lorazepam, zolpidem), muscle relaxants, narcotic pain relievers, psychiatric medications (e.g., nortriptyline, trazodone), and OTC cough and cold medications.
- Black cohosh with duloxetine may increase the risk of liver toxicity.
- Duloxetine with certain arrhythmia medications can increase the level of duloxetine or the other medication in the blood, which in turn increases your risk of side effects.

- Certain fluoroquinolone antibiotics can increase the level of duloxetine in your blood, which increases your risk of side effects.

Tell Your Doctor

- About any allergies you have, and all prescription and OTC medications you take, as well as supplements.
- If you have severe kidney disease or liver disease.
- If you have a personal or family history of psychiatric disorders (e.g., bipolar disorder, major depression), personal or family history of suicide attempts, diabetes, glaucoma, kidney disease, stomach problems, severe dehydration, drug or alcohol abuse, or seizure disorder.
- If you have diabetes, monitor your blood sugar levels regularly and inform your doctor of your results. Your doctor may need to adjust your medication, diet, and exercise when you begin or stop duloxetine.

Of Special Interest to Women

- In animal studies, duloxetine has had a negative impact on fetal development. Research also shows that babies born to women who used duloxetine during the last trimester may develop withdrawal symptoms such as seizures, muscle stiffness, constant crying, and feeding and/or breathing difficulties. Duloxetine should be used during pregnancy only if your physician determines the potential benefits justify the potential risk to the fetus.
- Duloxetine is excreted into breast milk. Because the impact of duloxetine on infants is not known, do not breast-feed while using this drug.
- Duloxetine may have a negative impact on your sex drive and/or ability to have an orgasm.

Symptoms of Overdose

Agitation, confusion, fainting, hallucinations, nausea, seizures, and vomiting.

Escitalopram

Brand Name

Lexapro

Available as Generic?

No

Principal Uses

Depression, generalized anxiety disorder

About the Drug

Escitalopram is a selective serotonin reuptake inhibitor, a drug class that includes citalopram (Celexa), fluoxetine (Prozac), paroxetine (Paxil), and sertraline (Zoloft). Escitalopram and other SSRIs affect brain chemicals called neurotransmitters, which the nerves use to send messages to each other. Neurotransmitters are produced and released by nerves and then travel to other nerves, where they attach to receptors.

Some neurotransmitters do not attach themselves to receptors and are taken up by the nerves that produced them. This action is called "reuptake," and it results in an imbalance of neurotransmitters, which is believed to be a cause of depression. Escitalopram prevents the reuptake of the neurotransmitter serotonin, which results in more serotonin being available to the brain to bind to receptors. Therefore, it helps restore the balance of neurotransmitters in the brain and improves feelings of well-being and energy level, as well as decreases nervousness.

How to Use This Drug

Escitalopram is available as tablets and liquid. This drug should be taken once daily in the morning or evening, with or without food. The usual starting dose for the tablets is 10 mg once daily, which may be increased to 20 mg after 1 week. A daily dose of 20 mg may not be any more beneficial than 10 mg daily for treatment of depression, so always strive for the lowest effective dose.

If you use the liquid, measure the dose prescribed by your physician using the special measuring device that comes with the prescription. Do not use a kitchen spoon.

It is typical not to feel any benefit from escitalopram for 1–2 weeks and not to feel the full benefit for up to 4 weeks after starting treatment.

Never take escitalopram that has been purchased on the Internet or from sources outside the United States. Investigators have found some samples of escitalopram purchased on the Internet to contain haloperidol (Haldol), a potent antipsychotic that has serious side effects.

Side Effects

- Common side effects: agitation or restlessness, blurry vision, decreased sexual desire or ability, diarrhea, drowsiness, dry mouth, fever, frequent urination, headache, indigestion, increased or decreased appetite, increased sweating, nausea, sleep difficulties, taste changes, tremors, and weight changes.
- Escitalopram may increase the risk of suicide in individuals age 24 and younger.

- Rare but serious side effects: bloody or tarry stools, change in the amount or urine, easy bruising or bleeding, fainting, irregular or pounding heartbeat, muscle weakness or cramps, stomach pain, tremor, or vomit that looks like coffee grounds.
- Withdrawal symptoms may occur when stopping escitalopram. They include dizziness, irritability, poor mood, tingling, tiredness, and vivid dreams. To avoid these symptoms, the dose of escitalopram should be reduced gradually.
- Serotonin syndrome may occur when you start or increase the dose of this drug. Seek immediate medical attention if you develop fast heartbeat, hallucinations, loss of coordination, restlessness, severe dizziness, severe nausea, vomiting and/or diarrhea, twitchy muscles, or unexplained fever.

Possible Drug, Supplement, and/or Food Interactions

- Escitalopram with aspirin, diclofenac, ibuprofen, indomethacin, nabumetone, naproxen, piroxicam, and other medications to treat arthritis, fever, pain, or swelling may cause you to bleed or bruise easily, or increase the risk of gastrointestinal bleeding.
- Drinking alcohol may increase some of the side effects of escitalopram.
- Sleeping pills, muscle relaxants, cold or allergy medications, narcotics, and medications for seizures or anxiety may increase the sleepiness caused by escitalopram.
- The following drugs may interact with escitalopram; you should talk to your doctor before using them: carbamazepine (Tegretol), cimetidine (Tagamet), lithium (Lithobid), warfarin (Coumadin), amitriptyline (Elavil), citalopram (Celexa), fluoxetine (Prozac), fluvoxamine (Luvox), imipramine (Tofranil), nortriptyline (Pamelor), paroxetine (Paxil), sertraline (Zoloft), almotriptan (Axert), sumatriptan (Imitrex), naratriptan (Amerge), or zolmitriptan (Zomig).
- Escitalopram should not be taken with MAOIs such as isocarboxazid (Marplan), phenelzine (Nardil), or selegiline (Eldepryl). Wait at least 14 days after stopping an MAOI before taking escitalopram. After you stop taking escitalopram, wait at least 14 days before you start taking an MAOI.
- Escitalopram (or any SSRI) with tryptophan can cause dizziness, headache, nausea, and sweating.

Tell Your Doctor

- If you have any allergies, and and all prescription and OTC medications you take, as well as supplements.

- If you have liver disease, kidney disease, seizures or epilepsy, bipolar disorder, stomach bleeding, dehydration, low sodium in the blood, or a history of drug abuse or suicidal thoughts.
- Immediately if you experience any new or worsening symptoms, such as mood or behavior changes, aggression, hostility, restlessness, hyperactivity, increased depression, anxiety, panic attacks, difficulty sleeping, or thoughts of suicide or harming yourself.

Of Special Interest to Women

- Escitalopram is in FDA pregnancy Category C, which means it may cause serious or life-threatening lung problems in infants. If you are planning to get pregnant or are pregnant and are taking escitalopram, talk to your health-care provider immediately to see if you should keep taking it or switch to another treatment for your depression or anxiety.
- Do not breast-feed if you are using escitalopram, because it passes into breast milk and can harm an infant.
- If you are elderly, you may be more sensitive to the effects of escitalopram. This drug may cause you to lose too much salt, especially if you are also taking diuretics.

Symptoms of Overdose

Coma, confusion, dizziness, nausea, rapid heartbeat, sweating, tremors, and vomiting.

Esomeprazole

Brand Name

Nexium

Available as Generic?

No

Principal Uses

Stomach and duodenal ulcers, gastroesophageal reflux disease (GERD)

About the Drug

Esomeprazole is a proton pump inhibitor, which means it blocks the action of the enzyme in the stomach wall that produces stomach acid. Once the enzyme is blocked, acid production is reduced, and the stomach and esophagus are able to heal.

In addition to being prescribed for GERD, esomeprazole is used along with amoxicillin and clarithromycin for treating ulcers and infection with the bacteria *H. pylori*. If you are taking NSAIDs on a regular basis, your doctor may suggest that you take esomeprazole because it can reduce the risk of gastric ulcers associated with long-term NSAID use.

How to Use This Drug

Esomeprazole is available in capsules and a delayed-release oral suspension, and it can be given intravenously. The capsules should be taken 1 hour before meals and swallowed whole. If you cannot swallow the capsule, you can open it and mix the pellets with pudding or applesauce. Do not chew the pellets.

A typical dose of esomeprazole to treat GERD is 20 or 40 mg taken once daily for 4–8 weeks. To help prevent NSAID-induced ulcers, the dose is 20–40 mg daily for 6 months. If you are treating *H. pylori* infection, 40 mg once daily along with amoxicillin and clarithromycin for 10 days is the normal course.

The delayed-release oral suspension can be taken by mouth. Mix the contents of the medication packet with 1 tablespoon of water and mix well. Let it sit for 2–3 minutes to thicken and consume it within 30 minutes. Do not chew or crush the granules because this may destroy the drug and/or increase the chances of experiencing side effects. You can take antacids along with esomeprazole if necessary.

Side Effects

- Common side effects: diarrhea, dizziness, dry mouth, headache, nausea, rash, and vomiting.
- Less common side effects: abnormal heartbeat, leg cramps, muscle pain, nervousness, and water retention.
- Unlikely but serious side effects: severe abdominal pain, persistent nausea and vomiting, dark urine, jaundice, and signs of vitamin B_{12} deficiency in people who take this medication for longer than 3 years (e.g., sore tongue, numbness or tingling of the hands and feet, and unusual weakness).

Possible Drug, Supplement, and/or Food Interactions

- Esomeprazole can increase the concentration of diazepam (Valium) by decreasing the elimination of diazepam in the liver.
- Esomeprazole can reduce the absorption and concentration in blood of ketoconazole (Nizoral). This may reduce the effectiveness of ketoconazole.
- Esomeprazole can increase the absorption and concentration in blood of digoxin (Lanoxin). This can increase digoxin toxicity.
- Blood levels of saquinavir (Invirase) may rise when used with esomeprazole.

- Blood levels of nelfinavir (Viracept) and atazanavir (Reyataz) may be reduced when used with esomeprazole.
- Esomeprazole reduces the activity of enzymes that convert clopidogrel (Plavix) to its active form in the liver.
- Esomeprazole increases the concentration of cilostazol (Pletal) and its metabolites, which means your doctor will likely reduce your cilostazol dose if you are also taking esomeprazole.
- Iron and calcium supplements need an adequate amount of stomach acid to be absorbed properly. Because esomeprazole reduces stomach acid, you may need to change the amount you take of these supplements or eat more foods rich in these nutrients.

Tell Your Doctor
- If you are allergic to esomeprazole or similar drugs (e.g., lansoprazole, omeprazole), or if you have any other allergies.
- About all prescription and OTC medications you are taking, as well as supplements.
- If you have a history of liver disease and/or stomach problems.
- Immediately if you experience heartburn along with dizziness, sweating, light-headedness, chest pain, shoulder or jaw pain, difficulty breathing, pain that spreads to the arms and shoulders, and unexplained weight loss.

Of Special Interest to Women
- No adequate evaluations of the effects of esomeprazole have been done in pregnant or nursing women. Based on information for similar drugs, however, esomeprazole may pass into breast milk.

Symptoms of Overdose
Confusion, blurry vision, extreme sweating, and rapid heartbeat.

Etanercept

Brand Name
Enbrel

Available as Generic?
No

Principal Uses
Rheumatoid arthritis, plaque psoriasis, psoriatic arthritis, ankylosing spondylitis, juvenile idiopathic arthritis

About the Drug

Etanercept belongs to a class of medications called biological response modifiers (BRMs), or biologics for short.

People who have inflammatory diseases such as rheumatoid arthritis and the others listed above have too much tumor necrosis factor (TNF) in their bodies. TNF is made by the body's immune system. Etanercept works with the immune system to reduce the levels of active TNF in the body. Because etanercept suppresses the immune system, it places users at great risk for developing serious infections.

If you have rheumatoid arthritis, you may use etanercept along with methotrexate if you do not get enough relief from methotrexate alone. For psoriatic arthritis, etanercept can prevent progressive destruction of the joints as well as improve physical function.

How to Use This Drug

Etanercept comes as three components: a solution in a prefilled syringe, an automatic injection device, and a powder that you mix with the solution. After you receive your first injection at your doctor's office, he or she can instruct you or another individual who may be administering your medication how to inject the medication under the skin. The typical treatment is 1 or 2 injections per week (25 mg per dose), but follow the directions provided by your doctor.

Inject the drug at different sites each time to reduce the chances of soreness and redness. Typical injection sites are the front of the thighs, the outer part of the upper arms, and the stomach except the navel and the region 2 inches around it. If you are treating psoriasis, do not inject the medication into skin that is red, raised, scaly, or thick.

Often physicians start patients who have chronic plaque psoriasis on higher doses and then decrease the dose after 3 months when the condition is under control.

Before injecting etanercept, look at the solution to make sure it is clear and colorless and that the expiration date has not passed. The solution may contain small white particles, which is usually safe, but do not use solution that contains colored or large particles or that is cloudy.

A vial of etanercept may contain enough medication for more than one dose. You can store vials of etanercept for up to 14 days after you have mixed the solution. However, never combine the contents of two or more vials to make a complete dose.

Side Effects

- Common side effects: reactions at the injection site (e.g., redness, swelling, itching, bruising, in up to 37% of patients), headache (17%), runny or irritated nose (12%), dizziness (7%), sore throat (7%), and cough (6%).

- Less common side effects: general weakness (5%), abdominal pain (5%), breathing problems (5%), heartburn (4%), vomiting (3%), and mouth ulcers (2%).

- A significant concern regarding etanercept is a decreased ability to fight infection from bacteria, viruses, and fungi, which increases your risk of developing a mild, moderate, serious, or life-threatening infection, including sepsis (an infection that affects the entire body) (see "Tell Your Doctor" below). Up to 34% of users develop an infection, such as the common cold or a sinus infection.

- Contact your doctor immediately if you experience any of the following symptoms during or shortly after your treatment: weakness, sweating, breathing difficulties, sore throat, cough, fever, flulike symptoms, fatigue, seizures, bruising, rash or hives, vision problems, dizziness, numbness or tingling, blistering skin, red or painful skin, or other signs of infection.

- Etanercept may increase the risk of developing leukemia.

Possible Drug, Supplement, and/or Food Interactions

- Etanercept may interact with vaccines for chicken pox, MMR, polio, rotavirus, smallpox, yellow fever, BCG (used in some countries for tuberculosis), and the nasal form of FluMist (the injected vaccine is not live).

- Etanercept with anakinra (Kineret) or abatacept (Orencia) can increase your chance of getting an infection.

- Etanercept with cyclophosphamide (Cytoxan) can increase the risk of developing tumors.

Tell Your Doctor

- About any allergies you have, and all prescription and OTC medications you take, as well as supplements.

- Because of the increased risk of infection associated with use of this drug, tell your doctor if you have any type of infection, including minor ones (e.g., open cuts or sores), cold sores, and chronic infections.

- If you have diabetes or any condition that affects the immune system, or if you have ever had seizures, a nervous system disease (e.g., multiple sclerosis), traverse myelitis (inflammation of the spinal cord), optic neuritis (inflammation of the optic nerve), blood abnormalities, hepatitis B, or heart failure.

- If you are taking medications that reduce the ability of the immune system to fight infections, such as abatacept (Orencia), azathioprine

(Imuran), cancer chemotherapy drugs, cyclophosphamide (Cytoxan), cyclosporine (Sandimmune), oral corticosteroids, methotrexate (Rheumatrex), sirolimus (Rapamune), sulfasalazine (Azulfidine), and tacrolimus (Prograf).

- If you are pregnant, plan to become pregnant, or are breast-feeding.
- Before having any vaccinations if you are using etanercept.
- Immediately if you are exposed to chicken pox while using etanercept.
- If you have ever lived in an area where severe fungal infections are common, including the Ohio and Mississippi river valleys.
- Etanercept increases the risk of developing tuberculosis, especially if you are already infected but do not have any symptoms. Your doctor may perform a TB test to see if you have an inactive TB infection.
- If you are using prefilled syringes or automatic injection devices, tell your doctor if you are allergic to latex. Do not let anyone who is allergic to latex inject you or handle the injection devices.

Of Special Interest to Women

- The FDA has classified etanercept as a pregnancy Category B medication, which means it does not appear to cause harm to the fetus based on animal studies. However, because animals do not always respond to medications in the same way that people do, the impact of etanercept on pregnant women is not known.
- It is not known whether etanercept is excreted in human breast milk. Therefore, it is not recommended for women who are breast-feeding.
- In rare cases, etanercept has caused autoimmune hepatitis or lupus-like conditions involving an unexplained rash across the cheeks and nose and ulcers in the nose and mouth. Symptoms of autoimmune hepatitis include stomach pain, jaundice, fatigue, loss of appetite, dark urine, and pale-colored stools.
- Etanercept can interfere with the results of certain lab tests, so be sure to let lab personnel know you are taking this medication.

Symptoms of Overdose

Not known, because there have been very few cases of patients taking too much of the drug. If you suspect you have taken an overdose, seek medical assistance as soon as possible.

Etonogestrel/Ethinyl Estradiol

Brand Name
NuvaRing

Available as Generic?

No

Principal Use

To prevent pregnancy

About the Drug

Etonogestrel and ethinyl estradiol is a combination of female hormones that prevents the release of an egg from an ovary (ovulation). This medication also causes your cervical mucus and uterine lining to change so it is more difficult for sperm to reach the uterus and for a fertilized egg to attach to the uterine wall.

How to Use This Drug

This medication comes with instructions; follow the directions carefully regarding insertion, replacement, and removal. Your doctor will tell you which day of your menstrual cycle to insert your first vaginal ring. You may need to use backup birth control (e.g., condoms, spermicide; not a diaphragm) during the first week you use your first vaginal ring.

Leave the ring in place for 3 full weeks. Remove the ring after 3 weeks, on the same day of the week you inserted it and at about the same time of day. Allow 1 full week to go by before you insert the new ring. Your menstrual period should begin during the week you are not wearing the vaginal ring. Insert the new ring on the same day of the week you inserted it in the last cycle, even if you are still menstruating.

It is critical that you follow the instructions provided with the vaginal ring and by your health-care provider to prevent pregnancy. If the vaginal ring falls out, rinse it with warm water and reinsert it. Do not leave the ring out for longer than 3 hours. Consult your health-care provider if you have any questions or concerns about your use of the vaginal ring. Call your doctor if you fail to follow the proper schedule of use.

Side Effects

- Most common side effects: appetite changes, bloating, breast pain, tenderness or swelling, decreased sex drive, dizziness, freckles or darkening of facial skin, hair loss (scalp), headache, increased body hair, menstrual changes, nausea (mild), stomach cramps, tiredness, vaginal itching or discharge, vomiting.
- Serious side effects: balance problems; breast lump; chest pain or a heavy feeling; confusion; dark urine; depression; low fever; nausea; pain behind the eyes; stomach pain; speech problems; swelling of the hands, ankles, or feet; sudden headache; sudden weakness or numbness; vision problems; yellowing of the skin or eyes.

Possible Drug, Supplement, and/or Food Interactions
- Some drugs may make etonogestrel and ethinyl estradiol less effective, which may result in pregnancy. Tell your doctor if you are taking acetaminophen, amobarbital, atazanavir, butabarbital, carbamazepine, felbamate, fosamprenavir, griseofulvin, indinavir, lopinavir, mephobarbital, modafinil, nelfinavir, oxcarbazepine, phenobarbital, phenytoin, primidone, rifampin, ritonavir, secobarbital, tipranavir, and topiramate.
- Ascorbic acid (vitamin C) and Saint-John's-wort may make etonogestrel and ethinyl estradiol less effective.

Tell Your Doctor
- About any allergies you have, and all prescription and OTC medications you take, as well as supplements.
- If you have a history of any of the following conditions, as you should not use this medication: stroke, blood clot, circulation problems, heart valve disorder, hormone-related cancer such as breast or uterine cancer, abnormal vaginal bleeding, liver disease, liver cancer, severe high blood pressure, migraine, jaundice caused by birth control pills.
- If you have any of the following conditions, because your doctor may need to adjust your dose or conduct tests before you can safely take etonogestrel and ethinyl estradiol: abnormal mammogram; angina; congestive heart failure; depression; diabetes; epilepsy or seizures; fibrocystic breast disease; gallbladder disease; history of heart attack; heart disease; high blood pressure; high cholesterol or triglycerides; irregular menstrual cycles; kidney disease; migraine; prolapsed uterus, bladder, or rectum; severe constipation; toxic shock syndrome; vaginal irritation.

Of Special Interest to Women
- The vaginal ring can cause birth defects. Do not use it if you are pregnant or suspect you are pregnant. Contact your health-care provider immediately if you become pregnant while using the vaginal ring.
- The hormones in the vaginal ring can pass into breast milk and harm a nursing infant. Do not use this medication if you are breast-feeding.
- Taking hormones like those in the vaginal ring can increase your risk of blood clots, stroke, or heart attack, especially if you are older than 35 and if you smoke. Do not smoke while using the vaginal ring.
- The vaginal ring does not protect women against sexually transmitted diseases. You should use a condom to protect yourself against these diseases.
- Do not use a diaphragm as backup birth control, because the vaginal ring may hinder the correct placement and position of the diaphragm.

- Vaginal lubricants, yeast infection treatments, and spermicides should not jeopardize the integrity of the vaginal ring. However, discuss the use of other vaginal products with your health-care provider while using a vaginal ring.

Symptoms of Overdose

Nausea, vaginal bleeding, or vomiting.

Fish Oil Supplements

Brand Names

Various, including Carlson, Nature Made, Nordic Naturals, Schiff, Twinlab

Available as Generic?

Yes

Principal Uses

Inflammatory conditions such as rheumatoid arthritis, inflammatory bowel disease, and heart disease; also used to treat depression, lupus, osteoporosis

About the Supplement

Fish oil supplements contain omega-3 fatty acids, specifically eicosapentaenoic acid (EPA) and docosahexaenoic acid (DHA). Omega-3s are polyunsaturated fats that are essential for overall health, but because the body cannot produce them you must get them from food or supplements. These fats can be derived directly from certain foods, especially cold-water fatty fish such as halibut, herring, salmon, and tuna; less-rich sources are some plant and nut oils, including flaxseed, hemp, and walnuts.

Research suggests that the body may absorb omega-3 fatty acids better from food than from supplements. However, the majority of women do not get enough omega-3s in their diet, so a supplement can be a wise alternative not only to meet a healthy level of these fatty acids but also to treat a variety of health issues.

EPA has a role in the prevention of cardiovascular disease, and DHA is necessary for proper development and function of the brain and nervous system. In fact, omega-3 fatty acids are highly concentrated in the brain and seem to have an important role in cognitive and behavioral functioning. Studies also suggest that fish oil/omega-3 fatty acids are helpful in the prevention and/or treatment of high cholesterol, high blood pressure, heart disease, rheumatoid arthritis, lupus, osteoporosis, depression, menstrual pain, bipolar disorder, breast cancer, and colon cancer.

How to Use This Supplement

Base your selection of a fish oil supplement on the amount of EPA and DHA in the supplement, not on the total amount of fish oil. A typical amount to look for is 180–360 mg of EPA and 120–240 mg of DHA per capsule. The American Heart Association recommends taking 1 g daily of EPA and DHA if you have coronary heart disease, and 2–4 g daily if you have high cholesterol. Do not take more than 3 g daily of fish oil daily without consulting your health-care provider because there is an increased risk of bleeding at that dose.

Because of possible contamination of fish oils, purchase brands only from companies that state they have purified and tested their supplements to ensure they contain no mercury or pesticide residues.

Side Effects

- Most common side effects: belching, bloating, diarrhea, and gas.
- Fish oils can cause bruising or excessive bleeding if you tend to bruise easily or have a bleeding disorder.

Possible Drug, Supplement, and/or Food Interactions

- Use fish oil supplements with caution if you are taking blood-thinning medications such as clopidogrel or warfarin, because they can increase the risk of bleeding and/or bruising easily.
- Fish oil supplements may increase fasting blood sugar levels; consult your health-care provider if you are taking medications to lower blood sugar (e.g., glipizide, glyburide, insulin). Your doctor may need to adjust your dose.
- Fish oil supplements may reduce the toxic side effects (e.g., kidney damage, high blood pressure) associated with cyclosporine.
- If you are treating psoriasis with etretinate and topical corticosteroids, use of fish oils (especially EPA) may improve symptoms.
- Omega-3 fatty acids may reduce the risk of ulcers from use of NSAIDs.

Tell Your Doctor

- If you have any allergies, and all OTC and prescription medications you are taking, as well as supplements.
- If you are planning to take fish oil/omega-3 fatty acids.
- If you have any health issues that may require monitoring while you take the supplements, such as a bleeding disorder or use of other medications.

- If you are a vegetarian and do not eat fish. Ask your doctor if he or she can prescribe a different product.

Of Special Interest to Women
- Studies show that infants who did not get an adequate amount of omega-3 fatty acids from their mothers during pregnancy are at risk for developing nervous system problems and difficulties with vision.
- Although you should always look for fish oil supplements that are not contaminated, this is especially important if you are pregnant or breast-feeding. Choose fish oil supplements that have been purified and tested for toxins. You may also choose an omega-3 fatty acid supplement that is not derived from fish. Talk to your health-care provider about taking DHA derived from algae.
- Fish oil supplements can help reduce triglyceride levels, a risk factor for heart disease that is especially important for women who are taking hormone therapy.

Symptoms of Overdose
Upset stomach, as well as a severe case of any of the common side effects. Excessive internal bleeding is also a possibility.

Fluoxetine

Brand Names
Prozac, Sarafem
Available as Generic?
Yes
Principal Uses
Depression, bulimia, obsessive-compulsive disorder, panic disorder, premenstrual dysphoric disorder
About the Drug
Fluoxetine is an SSRI, a drug class that includes citalopram (Celexa), paroxetine (Paxil), and sertraline (Zoloft). Fluoxetine affects the activity of the neurotransmitter serotonin, which facilitates communication among nerves in the brain. A commonly held theory about a cause of depression is that it is related to an imbalance among neurotransmitters. Fluoxetine prevents the reuptake of serotonin, which increases the amount of free serotonin available in the brain to stimulate nerve cells. This action in turn may improve mood, sleep, appetite, and energy levels, as well as decrease anxiety, panic attacks, compulsions, obsessions, and bingeing and purging behaviors.

How to Use This Drug

Fluoxetine is available in tablets, capsules (traditional and long-acting), and solution. It can be taken with or without food. Fluoxetine (Prozac) is usually taken once daily in the morning or twice daily in the morning and at noon. The delayed-release formula is usually taken once a week.

The typical dose for treatment of depression is 20–80 mg daily. Bulimia is usually treated with 60 mg daily, obsessive-compulsive disorder with 20–60 mg daily, and panic disorder with 10–60 mg daily. For premenstrual dysphoric disorder, fluoxetine (Sarafem) is typically taken once daily, either every day or on certain days of the month, usually the 2 weeks before your period through the first full day of your period.

If you use the liquid form of fluoxetine, measure the dose using the special measuring device provided with your prescription. It usually takes 2 or more weeks to feel the full benefits of fluoxetine.

Side Effects

- Common side effects: anxiety, drowsiness, headache, insomnia, loss of appetite, and nausea.
- Less likely but serious side effects: blurry vision, increased blood pressure, seizures, severe skin rashes, sexual dysfunction, shakiness, uncontrolled movements, unusual mental/mood changes, and vasculitis (inflammation of small blood vessels).
- Rare but very serious side effects that you should report immediately to your doctor: black stools, changes in the amount of urine, easy bruising or bleeding, fainting, fast/irregular heartbeat, muscle weakness or spasm, seizures, and vomit that looks like coffee grounds.
- Symptoms of withdrawal include anxiety, insomnia, nausea, and nervousness. Ask your doctor how to safely taper off the drug.
- Antidepressants, including fluoxetine, may increase the risk of suicidal thinking and behavior in young people (up to age 25) during the early treatment period. Contact your health-care provider immediately if you experience these side effects.
- Rarely, fluoxetine can cause serotonin syndrome, and the risk increases if you take fluoxetine with certain other drugs (see "Possible Drug, Supplement, and/or Food Interactions"). Seek immediate medical attention if you experience fast heartbeat, fever, hallucinations, loss of coordination, severe dizziness, severe nausea/vomiting/diarrhea, or twitchy muscles.

Possible Drug, Supplement, and/or Food Interactions

- Fluoxetine with any MAOIs, such as isocarboxazid (Marplan) or phenelzine (Nardil), may result in coma, confusion, high blood pressure, tremor, and death. Fluoxetine should not be taken for at least 14 days after stopping MAOIs, and MAOIs should not be taken for at least 5 weeks after stopping fluoxetine.

- Do not take drugs that increase serotonin levels without consulting your physician. These include bromocriptine, buspirone, dextromethorphan, lithium, meperidine, propoxyphene, phentermine, SSRIs, SNRIs, tryptophan, Saint-John's-wort, sumatriptan, and other "triptans."
- Fluoxetine with drugs that increase serotonin levels can cause a very serious condition called serotonin syndrome. These drugs include triptans (e.g., eletriptan, sumatriptan), SSRIs (e.g., citalopram, paroxetine), SNRIs (e.g., duloxetine, venlafaxine), lithium, tramadol, and tryptophan. Your risk of serotonin syndrome is greater whenever you start or increase the dose of any of these medications.
- Other drugs that can interact with fluoxetine include antianxiety drugs (e.g., alprazolam), antipsychotics (e.g., aripiprazole), antiarrhythmics (e.g., flecainide), carbamazepine, cimetidine, diuretics (e.g., furosemide), metoprolol, tricyclic antidepressants (e.g., imipramine).
- Fluoxetine with warfarin, NSAIDs, or other drugs that affect bleeding may increase your risk of upper gastrointestinal bleeding.

Tell Your Doctor
- If you have any allergies and all OTC and prescription medications you are taking, as well as supplements.
- If you have a personal or family history of bipolar disorder or suicide attempts, liver problems, dehydration, seizures, or gastrointestinal ulcers.
- If you have diabetes or alcohol dependence. The liquid form of fluoxetine may contain sugar or alcohol.

Of Special Interest to Women
- Do not take fluoxetine during pregnancy unless your health-care provider decides it is clearly needed. Fluoxetine during the third trimester may cause withdrawal symptoms in your infant, such as breathing and feeding difficulties, constant crying, muscle stiffness, and seizures.
- Fluoxetine passes into breast milk and may cause undesirable effects. Therefore, it is not recommended to take fluoxetine while breast-feeding.

Symptoms of Overdose
Fainting, irregular heartbeat, seizures and severe dizziness.

Folic Acid

Brand Names

Various, including GNC, Jarrow Formulas, Nature Made, Nature's Bounty, Twinlab; also an ingredient in many combination vitamin products

Available as Generic?

Yes

Principal Use

Helps prevent birth defects such as spina bifida

About the Supplement

As a B vitamin, folic acid (also referred to as vitamin B_9) plays a major role in converting carbohydrates into glucose, which is then used by the body to produce energy. Folic acid is necessary for proper brain function and therefore has a significant role in mental and emotional health. It assists in the production of genetic material—DNA and RNA—and is instrumental in the growth of cells and tissues during infancy, adolescence, and pregnancy. Folic acid also has a role, along with vitamin B_{12}, in regulating the formation of red blood cells.

Folic acid is the synthetic form of vitamin B_9 and the form used in supplements and fortified foods; folate is the form of the vitamin that occurs naturally in foods.

How to Use This Supplement

Folic acid is available as tablets and in combination vitamin supplements, including B-complex supplements. If you are trying to get pregnant, you need to get 400–800 mcg of folic acid every day. Women who are 50 and older need 400 mcg of folic acid daily. Do not take more than 1000 mcg of folic acid per day without consulting your health-care provider.

Side Effects

- At recommended doses, side effects from folic acid are very rare.
- Very high doses can cause seizures, skin reactions, sleep problems, and stomach upset.
- More than 800 micrograms of folic acid per day may mask an underlying vitamin B_{12} deficiency. Talk to your doctor about this dosage.

Possible Drug, Supplement, and/or Food Interactions

- Folic acid interferes with the absorption of tetracycline. Separate your doses of folic acid and tetracycline by several hours.

- Drugs that reduce the body's ability to absorb folate and thus indicate you may need to take a folic acid supplement include antacids, antiseizure medications (e.g., carbamazepine, phenytoin), proton pump inhibitors, bile acid sequestrants (e.g., cholestyramine, colestipol), birth control medications, NSAIDs, sulfasalazine, and triamterene.
- Methotrexate reduces the amount of folic acid in your body. If you take methotrexate, you may need to take folic acid supplements. However, do not take folic acid supplements without consulting your health-care provider.

Tell Your Doctor
- If you are planning to get pregnant or are pregnant, or if you are breast-feeding. Some doctors prescribe prenatal vitamins that contain higher amounts of folic acid than the 400–800 mcg typically recommended.
- If you have given birth to a baby with a birth defect of the spine or brain and you want to get pregnant again. Your health-care provider may prescribe high levels of folic acid before and during pregnancy to reduce your risk of having another baby with these conditions.
- If you have a family member who has spina bifida. Your doctor may prescribe a high level of folic acid for you before and during pregnancy.
- If you are taking medications to treat asthma, diabetes, epilepsy, inflammatory bowel disease, lupus, psoriasis, or rheumatoid arthritis, as you may need to take additional folic acid.
- If you have liver disease, sickle-cell disease, celiac disease, or kidney disease and are on dialysis.

Of Special Interest to Women
- Getting enough folic acid is especially important for women before and during pregnancy to help prevent major birth defects such as spina bifida and anencephaly. Some studies suggest that folic acid may help prevent other types of birth defects as well.
- Too little folic acid (or folate from foods) can result in anemia. Good sources of folate include leafy green vegetables; fruits; dried beans, peas, and nuts. Enriched breads and cereals also contain folic acid.

Symptoms of Overdose
Folic acid is a water-soluble vitamin, which means the body automatically eliminates it regularly. However, high doses of folic acid for a prolonged

period may cause bitter taste in the mouth, digestive problems, insomnia, irritability, rash, and zinc deficiency. Overdoses may also mask signs of a vitamin B_{12} deficiency, which can cause nerve damage, or increase the risk of heart attack in people who have heart disease.

Furosemide

Brand Names
  Delone, Lasix
Available as Generic?
  Yes
Principal Uses
  Controlling high blood pressure and treating water retention (edema) related to congestive heart failure, kidney failure, and cirrhosis
About the Drug
  Furosemide is a diuretic (water pill) and, more specifically, a loop diuretic, which means it affects a certain part of the kidneys known as the loop of Henle. The drug works by blocking the absorption of salt (sodium and chloride) and water from the fluid in the kidneys, which in turn increases the output of urine. As the amount of water in the blood declines, blood volume decreases, and blood pressure is lowered. Water retention also is improved.
How to Use This Drug
  Furosemide is available in tablets and as an injection. The oral drug begins to work within 1 hour after taking a dose, and the increase in urine output lasts for about 6–8 hours. If you receive an injection, the drug begins to work in 5 minutes and urine output increases for about 2 hours.
  The usual starting oral dose for high blood pressure is 40 mg twice daily. For edema, the starting dose is 20–80 mg, with an equal or greater dose taken 6–8 hours later if needed. Furosemide can be taken with or without food once or twice daily, as determined by your doctor. It is recommended that you take this medication at least 4 hours before bedtime to avoid having to get up to urinate during the night. Take furosemide at the same time each day.
Side Effects
  • Common side effects: dehydration, electrolyte depletion, and low blood pressure.

- Less common side effects: abdominal pain, diarrhea, dizziness, increased blood sugar and uric acid levels, jaundice, nausea, rash, ringing in the ears.
- Furosemide may cause an excessive loss of water and minerals. Let your doctor know immediately if you experience serious symptoms of dehydration such as muscle cramps or weakness, confusion, severe dizziness, unusual dry mouth or thirst, nausea or vomiting, irregular heartbeat, fainting, or seizures.
- Furosemide may make you more sensitive to sunlight. Wear protective clothing and sunscreen while taking furosemide.

Possible Drug, Supplement, and/or Food Interactions

Furosemide is known to interact with more than 600 drugs; however, most of the interactions are mild to moderate.

- Major interactions may occur with amikacin, amiodarone, bisacodyl/sodium biphosphate/sodium phosphate, cisapride, dofetilide, dolasetron, dronedarone, droperidol, gentamicin, kanamycin, levomethadyl acetate, lithium, neomycin, netilmicin, pimazide, tizanidine, tobramycin, and ziprasidone.
- Furosemide with aminoglycoside antibiotics (e.g., gentamicin) or the diuretic ethacrynic acid may cause hearing damage.
- Furosemide may interact with OTC cold and cough medications, pain/fever medications, and diet aids, including NSAIDs such as ibuprofen.
- Sucralfate, cholestyramine, and colestipol reduce the action of furosemide. They should be taken at least 2 hours apart from furosemide.
- Furosemide and aspirin may cause aspirin toxicity.

Tell Your Doctor

- If you have any allergies and all OTC and prescription medications you are taking, as well as supplements.
- If you have kidney disease, liver disease, lupus, or gout.
- If you have diabetes, because furosemide can impact blood sugar levels, and your doctor may need to adjust your diabetes medication and/or diet.

Of Special Interest to Women

- No adequate studies of the impact of furosemide on pregnant women have been done. Discuss the risks and benefits of using furosemide during pregnancy with your doctor.
- Furosemide is secreted into breast milk; therefore, avoid breastfeeding while taking this drug.

- Furosemide may reduce the potassium levels in your blood. Talk to your doctor about adding potassium to your diet or taking a potassium supplement while using furosemide.

Symptoms of Overdose

Fainting, a severe decrease in urination, and severe weakness.

Gabapentin

Brand Name

Neurontin

Available as Generic?

Yes

Principal Uses

Seizures and seizure disorders, nerve damage from shingles and postherpetic neuralgia; off-label use includes fibromyalgia, diabetic neuropathy, hot flashes, restless leg syndrome, headache

About the Drug

Gabapentin is an anticonvulsant that works by increasing the amount of the chemical gamma-aminobutyric acid (GABA) in the brain. If you use it to control seizures, it continues to be effective only as long as you take the drug. Gabapentin is also used to manage neuropathic pain conditions, but it is not effective for routine pain associated with arthritis or minor injuries. Research supported by the National Institutes of Health have found gabapentin effective in treating symptoms associated with fibromyalgia. Although the drug does not have FDA approval for this syndrome, some health-care providers prescribe it for this purpose.

How to Use This Drug

Gabapentin is available in tablets, capsules, and solution, and can be taken with or without food, as directed by your doctor. To minimize side effects, take your first dose at bedtime. Gabapentin works best when taken at evenly spaced intervals throughout the day and night.

Do not stop taking gabapentin without consulting your physician, so he or she can help you gradually decrease your dose.

Side Effects

- Most common side effects: constipation, dizziness, dry mouth, drowsiness, fatigue, nausea, unsteadiness, vision changes, and weight gain.
- Less likely but serious side effects: abdominal pain, breathing difficulties, depression, fast or irregular heartbeat, hearing loss, pain or red-

ness of the arms or legs, persistent sore throat/fever/cough, shaking or tremor, suicidal thoughts or attempts, swollen arms or legs, unusual bleeding or bruising.

Possible Drug, Supplement, and/or Food Interactions

- Antacids that contain aluminum or magnesium may interfere with the absorption of gabapentin. Take gabapentin at least 2 hours after taking an antacid.
- Gabapentin can affect the results of certain lab tests for protein levels in urine. Inform your doctor and lab personnel that you are using this drug before undergoing such lab tests.
- Gabapentin adds to the effects of alcohol and other substances that depress the central nervous system and make you drowsy or less alert, including antihistamines, sedatives, tranquilizers, prescription pain medications or narcotics, muscle relaxants, and anesthetics, including those used by dentists.

Tell Your Doctor

- If you have any allergies and all OTC and prescription medications you are taking, as well as supplements.
- If you have a history of kidney, liver, or heart disease.
- Immediately if you notice new or worsening symptoms such as mood or behavior changes, depression, anxiety, hostility, or hyperactivity.
- Gabapentin may cause suicidal thoughts during the first few months of treatment or whenever your doctor changes your dose. Contact your health-care provider immediately if you experience worsening depression or suicidal thoughts.

Of Special Interest to Women

- Gabapentin is an FDA Category C substance, which means it is not known whether it can harm the fetus. Use gabapentin during pregnancy only if your doctor clearly believes the benefits outweigh the risks.
- Gabapentin is excreted into breast milk, so consult your health-care provider before breast-feeding.
- Wear a medical alert bracelet or carry an ID card stating you are taking gabapentin in case of emergency. This is especially important if you are pregnant, require emergency medical care, and are unable to inform medical personnel about your medication use.

Symptoms of Overdose

Severe drowsiness, slurred speech, blurry vision, diarrhea, and extreme lethargy.

Glatiramer

Brand Name

Copaxone

Available as Generic?

No

Principal Use

To treat and prevent relapse of multiple sclerosis

About the Drug

Glatiramer is a combination of four amino acids (protein) that simulate myelin protein (the protective coating on nerve fibers in the brain and spinal cord). The drug appears to block T cells that damage the myelin, although experts are not sure exactly how the drug accomplishes this. In clinical trials, glatiramer significantly reduced the annual relapse rate and also reduced the development of new lesions in patients who had multiple sclerosis when compared with controls who received placebo. Glatiramer does not cure multiple sclerosis.

Glatiramer has been approved by the FDA to reduce the frequency of relapses in patients who have relapsing-remitting multiple sclerosis as well as for those who have had their first clinical episode of the disease.

How to Use This Drug

Glatiramer is given by injection under the skin, with the preferred sites being the abdomen, arms, thighs, and hips. You will be instructed by a health-care professional how to administer your own injections at home. The medication is available in vials and prefilled syringes that are designed for single use only. Dispose of the vial or syringe properly after each injection. Glatiramer can be stored in the refrigerator or kept at room temperature away from high heat, light, or moisture. Glatiramer will keep for up to 30 days if stored at room temperature. If you refrigerate glatiramer, warm it to room temperature before use.

Do not use glatiramer if the prefilled syringe appears cloudy or contains particles. Call your doctor for a new prescription.

Side Effects

- Up to 20% of patients experience reactions from the injection, which may include feeling anxious or experiencing a pounding heartbeat, tightness in the throat, or breathing difficulties. These reactions may occur even if you have been getting injections for some time.

- Less serious side effects: diarrhea, dizziness, joint pain, muscle tension or stiffness, nausea, urge to urinate, or white patches or sores inside your mouth or on your lips.
- Side effects associated at the injection site are very common and include redness (43%), pain (40%), itching (27%), a hard lump where the injection is given (26%), swelling (19%), and inflammation (9%).
- Serious side effects: chest pain, fast heart rate, flulike symptoms (fever, body aches, chills), and severe pain at the injection site.

Possible Drug, Supplement, and/or Food Interactions

- Glatiramer with natalizumab increases the risk of infections, including progressive multifocal leukoencephalopathy, a severe, debilitating, and potentially fatal viral infection that attacks the brain.
- Results from existing clinical trials do not suggest any significant drug interactions associated with glatiramer and other therapies typically used by patients who have multiple sclerosis, including the use of corticosteroids for up to 28 days. However, use of glatiramer has not been thoroughly evaluated in combination with interferon beta.

Tell Your Doctor

- If you have any allergies, especially to glatiramer and mannitol, and all OTC and prescription medications you are taking, as well as supplements.
- If you have heart disease.

Of Special Interest to Women

- Glatiramer is a pregnancy Category B medication, which means even though no adverse effects have been observed in animal studies, adequate studies have not been conducted in pregnant women. Therefore, you and your health-care provider should discuss the risks and benefits of using glatiramer during pregnancy.
- It is not known whether glatiramer is excreted into breast milk. Consult your physician if you want to breast-feed while taking glatiramer.

Symptoms of Overdose

Not known.

Glucosamine and Chondroitin

Brand Names

Various, including Cosamin, Doctor's Best, Nature Made, Puritan's Pride, Schiff, Sundown

Available as Generic?

Yes

Principal Uses

Arthritis, back pain, inflammation, temporomandibular joint disorder

About the Supplement

Glucosamine is a natural amino sugar that the body produces and distributes in cartilage and other connective tissue. As a supplement, glucosamine is most often made from the covering of shellfish, which contains glucosamine, but products made from corn are also available for individuals who are allergic to shellfish. Glucosamine supplements are available as glucosamine hydrochloride, N-acetyl-glucosamine (NAG), and glucosamine sulfate, which is the most common form.

Chondroitin is also found naturally in healthy cartilage and is a complex carbohydrate that helps cartilage retain water. The supplement forms are usually made from shark or bovine cartilage. Chondroitin is also known as chondroitin sulfate, chondroitin sulfuric acid, and chonsurid.

Some experts say glucosamine sulfate works by strengthening cartilage and facilitating the synthesis of glycoaminoglycans, a major ingredient in cartilage. Many people take the glucosamine and chondroitin combination, although glucosamine may be taken separately as well. Although these supplements are popular alternative treatments for osteoarthritis pain, results of numerous studies offer conflicting evidence concerning their effectiveness in reducing pain, inflammation, or joint destruction.

How to Use This Supplement

Glucosamine is available OTC as tablets, capsules, and liquid. The typical dose of glucosamine used in most published studies has been 500 mg three times daily or in one 1500 mg dose. When glucosamine is combined with chondroitin, the typical dose is 500 mg of glucosamine and 400 mg of chondroitin.

Side Effects

- Common side effects: drowsiness, gastrointestinal complaints, headache, insomnia, itching, leg pain, and sun sensitivity.
- Rare side effects: constipation, diarrhea, flatulence, heartburn, loss of appetite, nausea, and vomiting.
- Glucosamine may or may not alter blood sugar levels. If you have diabetes, exercise caution if taking glucosamine.

Possible Drug, Supplement, and/or Food Interactions

- The combination of glucosamine and chondroitin may increase the effects of warfarin.

- Glucosamine may increase the anti-inflammatory activity of NSAIDs such as ibuprofen, which may result in the need for lower doses of these drugs.

Tell Your Doctor
- If you have any allergies, especially to shellfish. Glucosamine supplements are often made from shellfish, so you will need to look for brands made from nonfish sources, such as corn.
- If you have diabetes. Your doctor may need to monitor your blood sugar levels or adjust your medication, as glucosamine may affect insulin levels and glucose metabolism.
- If you have any type of bleeding disorder. In theory, glucosamine may increase the risk of bleeding.
- If you are a vegetarian and do not want to take supplements that contain shark or bovine cartilage.
- If you are kosher and cannot take supplements that contain shellfish.

Of Special Interest to Women
- Do not use glucosamine and/or chondroitin while you are pregnant or breast-feeding. This is a precaution, because it is not known whether these supplements have any impact on fetal or infant health.

Symptoms of Overdose
Diarrhea or nausea.

Hydrochlorothiazide

Brand Names
Ezide, HydroDiuril, Hydro-Par, Microzide, and many combinations with other drugs

Available as Generic?
Yes

Principal Uses
High blood pressure, fluid accumulation

About the Drug
Hydrochlorothiazide is a diuretic (water pill) used to treat high blood pressure and the accumulation of fluid caused by cirrhosis, chronic kidney failure, use of corticosteroid medications, heart failure, and nephrotic syndrome. The drug works by blocking the reabsorption of salt and fluid by the kidneys, which results in an increase in urination. It is also used to treat kidney stones that contain calcium because it has the ability to reduce the amount of calcium excreted by

the kidneys and thus reduces the amount of calcium in urine available to form stones.

How to Use This Drug

Hydrochlorothiazide is available as tablets. It may be taken with or without food. The usual dose for high blood pressure is 12.5–50 mg once daily. For edema, the typical dose is 25–100 mg once daily or in divided doses.

To avoid having to get up often during the night to urinate, take your medication more than 4 hours before bedtime. Do not stop taking hydrochlorothiazide even when you feel well, as most people who have high blood pressure do not feel ill.

Side Effects

- Common side effects: blurry vision, constipation, diarrhea, dizziness, headache, increased sensitivity to sunlight, loss of appetite, reduced sexual function, and stomach upset.
- Less common and serious side effects: confusion, fainting, fast or irregular heartbeat, joint pain, muscle cramps, nausea, numbness or tingling of the arms or legs, seizures, severe dizziness, signs of infection (e.g., fever, persistent sore throat), thirst, dark urine, unusual decrease in the amount of urine, unusual drowsiness, very dry mouth, vomiting, weakness, yellowing of the skin or eyes.
- Hydrochlorothiazide can lower potassium, sodium, and magnesium levels. Your doctor may prescribe supplements or suggest dietary changes to prevent low levels of these minerals.

Possible Drug, Supplement, and/or Food Interactions

- Hydrochlorothiazide reduces the ability of the kidneys to eliminate lithium and can result in lithium toxicity.
- NSAIDs may reduce the ability of hydrochlorothiazide to lower blood pressure. This includes OTC medications such as ibuprofen and naproxen.
- Corticosteroids with hydrochlorothiazide can increase the risk for low levels of blood potassium and other electrolytes. Low blood potassium can increase the toxicity of digoxin.
- Cholestyramine and colestipol can reduce the ability of the gastrointestinal tract to absorb hydrochlorothiazide by up to 85%.
- Hydrochlorothiazide can have an influence on some lab tests. Tell your doctor and lab personnel that you are taking this drug before you undergo tests.

Tell Your Doctor

- If you have any allergies, especially to sulfa, as hydrochlorothiazide has a chemical structure similar to sulfa drugs.

- About all prescription and OTC medications you are taking, as well as supplements.
- If you have diabetes, as hydrochlorothiazide can raise blood sugar levels.
- If you have kidney disease, because hydrochlorothiazide can aggravate kidney dysfunction.
- If you have liver disease, untreated salt/mineral imbalance, dehydration, high cholesterol or triglycerides, gout, lupus, or recent nerve surgery.

Of Special Interest to Women
- No adequate studies of the impact of hydrochlorothiazide during pregnancy have been conducted. Consult your health-care provider about the benefits and risks associated with the use of hydrochlorothiazide during pregnancy.
- Hydrochlorothiazide is excreted in breast milk, and there is evidence that the drug can reduce production of breast milk as well. Discuss the risks and benefits of breast-feeding while using hydrochlorothiazide with your health-care provider.
- Hydrochlorothiazide can cause blood uric acid levels to rise, which may result in acute gout.
- Because hydrochlorothiazide may make you hypersensitive to sunlight, avoid prolonged exposure to the sun, tanning booths, and sunlamps. Wear protective clothing and sunscreen outdoors.

Symptoms of Overdose
Fainting, severe dizziness, and severe weakness.

Hydrocodone/Acetaminophen

Brand Names
Anexsia, Lorcet, Lorcet Plus, Norco, Vicodin, Vicodin ES
Available as Generic?
Yes
Principal Use
Chronic pain
About the Drug
The combination drug hydrocodone/acetaminophen was the most prescribed drug in the United States in 2009. For women who suffer with any type of chronic pain, this drug is often prescribed. Hydrocodone is a narcotic pain reliever and a cough suppressant that blocks the receptors on nerve cells in the brain that result in the sensation of pain. Acetaminophen

is a nonnarcotic pain reliever (analgesic) and fever reducer (antipyretic) that raises a person's threshold to pain and affects the temperature-regulating center of the brain.

How to Use This Drug

Hydrocodone/acetaminophen is available in tablets, capsules, and liquid. The usual dose for adults is 300–750 mg of acetaminophen and 2.5–10 mg of hydrocodone every 4–6 hours, or 15 mL of liquid every 4–6 hours as needed for pain.

Hydrocodone/acetaminophen can be taken with or without food. If you experience nausea, you can take it with food, but this may reduce the drug's effectiveness. This medication works best if taken before the pain becomes severe. Once the pain is intense, the medication is not as effective.

If you take hydrocodone/acetaminophen for an extended period of time, do not stop taking it suddenly without your doctor's approval. When this medication is taken for a prolonged period, it may not work as well, and your doctor may need to adjust your dose.

Side Effects

- Most frequent side effects: abnormally low blood pressure (which may make you feel light-headed), constipation, dizziness, sedation, nausea, vomiting.
- Less common: drowsiness; mood changes; vision changes; spasm of the ureter, which can make it difficult to urinate.
- Hydrocodone can impair your ability to think clearly.
- Hydrocodone can depress breathing and so should be used with caution if you are elderly, frail, or have a serious lung disease.
- Hydrocodone use can result in mental and physical dependence, but this is unlikely if you use this medication for short-term pain relief.
- Serious side effects that require immediate medical attention: slow or irregular breathing, slow or irregular heartbeat, a noticeable change in the amount of urine you excrete, and impaired or loss of hearing.
- Serious side effects associated with liver damage should be reported immediately to your doctor: severe nausea, yellowing of the eyes or skin, dark urine, stomach pain, extreme fatigue.

Possible Drug, Supplement, and/or Food Interactions

- Hydrocodone with alcohol and other sedatives can cause increased sedation and confusion.
- Carbamazepine with acetaminophen may increase the risk of liver toxicity.

- Be careful about taking hydrocodone with other medications for pain, cimetidine, isoniazid, MAO inhibitors, antiseizure drugs (e.g., carbamazepine, phenytoin), anticholinergics/antihistamines (e.g., hydroxyzine, oxybutynin, scopolamine), sedatives, tranquilizers, antianxiety drugs (e.g., diazepam), psychiatric medications (e.g., phenothiazines or tricyclics such as amitriptyline), muscle relaxants, antihistamines that cause drowsiness (e.g., diphenhydramine), or any combination medication that contains acetaminophen. Talk to your doctor about any of these combinations.

Tell Your Doctor
- If you have any allergies, especially to narcotics (e.g., morphine, codeine), and all OTC and prescription medications you are taking, as well as supplements.
- If you have severe breathing problems, severe diarrhea, difficulty urinating, liver disease, kidney disease, alcohol and/or drug dependency, heart problems, abdominal/stomach problems, lung disease, seizure disorders, serious head injury or brain disease, spinal problems, hypothyroidism, Addison's disease, or psychiatric problems.

Of Special Interest to Women
- Hydrocodone/acetaminophen is known to be excreted in breast milk, so nursing women should consult their doctor before using this medication.
- No adequate studies of hydrocodone/acetaminophen have been done in pregnant women. Talk to your doctor before using this drug if you are planning to get pregnant or are pregnant.

Symptoms of Overdose
Extreme fatigue, stomach pain, dark urine, yellowing of the eyes or skin, severe nausea, unusual sweating, vomiting, slowed breathing, slow heartbeat, cold and/or clammy skin, and loss of consciousness.

Ibandronate

Brand Name
Boniva
Available as Generic?
No
Principal Use
Prevent and treat osteoporosis in women after menopause

About the Drug

Ibandronate belongs to the class bisphosphonate, which includes alendronate, etidronate, risedronate, and zoledronic acid. Like all bisphosphonates, ibandronate prevents the breakdown of bone by bone cells called osteoclasts. Ibandronate can increase the amount of bone as well as bone strength, and reduce the risk of fractures.

How to Use This Drug

Ibandronate is available as tablets and as an intravenous (IV) injection. The oral dose can be taken once daily (2.5 mg) or once monthly (150 mg). Take monthly doses on the same day of each month. Take the tablets after rising and at least 60 minutes before eating or drinking anything (except plain water) or taking any other oral medications. This is important because absorption of ibandronate from the intestinal tract is poor, and food, beverages, or medications can further reduce absorption.

Swallow ibandronate tablets whole with 6–8 ounces of plain water while in an upright position to make sure the tablets enter the stomach and do not get caught in the esophagus. Never chew or suck on the tablets, as they can irritate the mouth and throat. Do not lie down for 60 minutes after taking ibandronate.

Ibandronate can also be administered intravenously at a dose of 3 mg every 3 months by a nurse or physician at a doctor's office or clinic. You and your doctor can discuss the best treatment plan for you.

Side Effects

- Most common side effects: abdominal pain, back pain, diarrhea, pain in the arms or legs, and redness or swelling of the eyes.
- Serious side effects are rare. Call your doctor if you experience chest pain; difficulty or pain when swallowing; new or worsening heartburn; pain or burning under the ribs or in the back; severe joint, bone, or muscle pain; jaw pain or numbness; black/tarry stools; or vomit that looks like coffee grounds.
- Severe irritation of the esophagus is an infrequent occurrence and should be reported to your doctor immediately.

Possible Drug, Supplement, and/or Food Interactions

- NSAIDs, including aspirin, can cause stomach irritation or ulcers. Talk to your doctor about how to safely use these drugs if you are taking ibandronate.
- Foods, beverages (except plain water), calcium and iron supplements, and medications can interfere with ibandronate absorption if taken before the oral dose or within 60 minutes after an oral dose.

- Ibandronate may affect the results of certain lab tests, so be sure to tell your doctor or lab personnel that you are taking this medication.

Tell Your Doctor
- If you have any allergies and all OTC and prescription drugs you are taking, as well as supplements.
- If you have low blood calcium levels (hypocalcemia) or severe kidney disease, or if you are not able to sit upright or stand for 60 minutes.
- If you have a history of disorders of the esophagus (e.g., esophageal stricture), difficulty swallowing, kidney problems, stomach and/or intestinal disorders (e.g., ulcers), anemia, or cancer.
- If you plan to have surgery, including dental surgery, tell your doctor or dentist that you are taking ibandronate. You may need to stop taking ibandronate before your procedure.
- If you have a vitamin D deficiency.

Of Special Interest to Women
- Ibandronate should be used during pregnancy only if your physician believes the potential benefits outweigh any potential risk to the fetus. Bisphosphonates have been shown to cause fetal damage in animals, but the risk to a human fetus is unknown.
- Ibandronate is passed into the breast milk of animals, but it is not known whether it appears in human breast milk. Do not breast-feed while taking ibandronate without discussing it with your physician.
- To make sure ibandronate is helping your condition, have your bone density checked regularly. You and your doctor can determine how often testing should be done.
- A literature review of ibandronate published in 2011 noted that 2.5 mg daily of oral ibandronate versus placebo reduced the incidence of new vertebral fractures by 62% over 3 years. Results of two other studies found that oral ibandronate 150 mg once monthly and 3 mg quarterly were superior to 2.5 mg daily in increasing bone mineral density over 2 years.

Symptoms of Overdose
Abdominal pain, diarrhea, heartburn, irritability, muscle cramps, numbness or tingling, seizures, tight muscles in the face, and unusual thoughts or behavior.

Ibuprofen

Brand Names
Advil, Medipren, Motrin, Nuprin

Available as Generic?

Yes

Principal Uses

Mild to moderate pain, fever, and inflammation, typically associated with arthritis, headache, menstrual cramps, and many other conditions

About the Drug

Ibuprofen is an NSAID, the drug class that includes aspirin, indomethacin, nabumetone, and naproxen. It is available by prescription and OTC. Pain, fever, and inflammation are promoted by chemicals called prostaglandins. Ibuprofen blocks the enzyme (cyclooxygenase) that makes prostaglandins, and the result is a reduction in the levels of prostaglandins.

How to Use This Drug

Ibuprofen is available in tablets, chewable tablets, capsules, oral drops, and oral suspension. Take ibuprofen with a full glass of water unless your doctor tells you otherwise. To avoid stomach upset, take ibuprofen with food. Do not lie down for at least 30 minutes after taking ibuprofen.

For mild to moderate pain, fever, menstrual cramps, and other minor pain conditions, the usual dose is 200 or 400 mg every 4–6 hours. For arthritis, the usual dose is 300–800 mg 3 or 4 times daily. When treating certain conditions, such as arthritis, it may take up to 2 weeks before you notice the full benefits of the drug. If you take ibuprofen on an as-needed basis, you can expect best results if you take it at the first signs of pain.

The maximum dose is 1.2 g daily unless you are under a doctor's care, and then the maximum dose is 3.2 g daily. Do not use ibuprofen for more than 10 days to treat pain or for more than 3 days to treat fever unless your doctor has given you other directions.

Side Effects

- Common side effects: constipation, diarrhea, dizziness, drowsiness, headache, heartburn, nausea, rash, ringing in the ears, upset stomach, and vomiting.
- Less common and serious side effects: difficult or painful swallowing, easy bruising or bleeding, rapid or pounding heartbeat, ringing in the ears, stomach pain, sudden or unexplained weight gain, swelling of the hands or feet, tarry or black stools, or vision changes. Contact your health-care provider immediately if these occur.
- Highly unlikely but very serious side effects: change in the amount of urine, dark urine, mental/mood changes, persistent sore throat or

fever, severe headache, unusual or extreme tiredness, very stiff neck, or yellowing of the skin or eyes. Contact your health-care provider immediately if any of these occur.

Possible Drug, Supplement, and/or Food Interactions

- Alcohol and/or smoking with ibuprofen can increase the risk of stomach bleeding.
- Ibuprofen may increase the blood levels of lithium, which can result in lithium toxicity.
- Ibuprofen may reduce the ability of blood pressure medications to lower blood pressure.
- Ibuprofen with aminoglycosides (e.g., gentamicin) may result in an elevated level of aminoglycosides in the blood and an increase in side effects.
- Do not use oral blood thinners or anticoagulants (e.g., warfarin) with ibuprofen because ibuprofen also thins the blood. Excessive blood thinning may result in bleeding and easy bruising.

Tell Your Doctor

- If you have any allergies, especially to aspirin or other NSAIDs, and all prescription and OTC medications you use, as well as supplements.
- If you have aspirin-sensitive asthma or recent heart bypass surgery, as you should not take ibuprofen.
- If you have had liver disease, poorly controlled diabetes, gastrointestinal problems (e.g., recurring heartburn, ulcers), heart disease, high blood pressure, stroke, swelling, dehydration, blood disorders, asthma, bleeding or clotting problems, or growths in the nose.
- If you have kidney disease or congestive heart failure, as ibuprofen can reduce the flow of blood to the kidneys and disrupt kidney function. This is most likely to occur if your kidney function is already impaired.

Of Special Interest to Women

- Ibuprofen should be used only when clearly necessary during the first 6 months of pregnancy. Do not use ibuprofen during the last 3 months because it can potentially result in premature closure of the ductus arteriosus in the fetal heart. The drug can also interfere with labor and delivery.
- Ibuprofen is not excreted in breast milk, so use of the drug while breast-feeding poses little risk to infants.

Symptoms of Overdose

Breathing difficulties, coffee ground–like vomit, extreme drowsiness, loss of consciousness, seizures, severe stomach pain, and unusually fast or slow heartbeat.

Infliximab

Brand Name

Remicade

Available as Generic?

No

Principal Uses

Rheumatoid arthritis, Crohn's disease, ankylosing spondylitis, psoriatic arthritis

About the Drug

Infliximab works by blocking the actions of tumor necrosis factor alpha (TNF alpha), which the body makes naturally. Blocking TNF alpha helps to reduce the inflammation associated with rheumatoid arthritis and other conditions for which this drug has been prescribed. This action also weakens the immune system, which can lead to serious side effects (see "Side Effects" below) while also slowing or stopping the damage caused by the disease being treated.

How to Use This Drug

Infliximab is given by intravenous injection over at least a 2-hour period by a health-care professional. Your doctor will determine the optimal dosage for your needs. After you receive your first treatment, the subsequent treatments are usually given again after 2 weeks, then 6 weeks, and then every 8 weeks thereafter, or as determined by your doctor.

Infliximab is prescribed either alone or combined with methotrexate when treating moderate to severe rheumatoid arthritis. It is typically used alone when treating other conditions indicated for this drug. The recommended dose for rheumatoid arthritis is 3 mg/kg as a single dose. For moderate to severe Crohn's disease, the dose is 5 mg/kg.

Side Effects

- Common side effects: abdominal pain, back pain, cough, fever, headache, nausea, upper respiratory tract infections, urinary tract infections, weakness, and vomiting.
- Less common and serious side effects: butterfly-shaped facial rash, chest pain, confusion, easy bruising/bleeding, joint pain, muscle

weakness, numbness/tingling of the arms and/or legs, pain/swelling at the injection site, shortness of breath, or swelling of the ankles/feet.

- Rarely, symptoms of liver disease may occur, including dark urine, extreme tiredness, severe abdominal pain, or yellowing of the eyes and/or skin.
- A decline in white and red blood cells and decreased platelet counts, as well as inflamed arteries (vasculitis), have been reported with infliximab.
- Your doctor may recommend being tested for tuberculosis before starting infliximab because the disease has been reactivated in people who have taken the drug.
- Infliximab is associated with an increased risk of infections.
- In rare cases, infliximab has caused multiple sclerosis, seizures, epilepsy, lupuslike conditions, and aplastic anemia.
- Infliximab may increase your risk of death if you have congestive heart disease. The drug also reportedly can worsen heart failure and cause new cases of heart failure.

Possible Drug, Supplement, and/or Food Interactions

The interaction of infliximab with other drugs has not been well explored. However, you should not start, stop, or change the dosage of any other medications you are taking without consulting your physician.

- Both anakinra and etanercept with infliximab can increase the risk of infection.
- Live vaccine (e.g., BCG for tuberculosis, nasal seasonal flu) should not be taken when using infliximab.
- Patients who use infliximab along with azathioprine or 6-mercaptopurine for the treatment of Crohn's disease have a very remote risk of developing hepatosplenic T-cell lymphoma.

Tell Your Doctor

- If you are allergic to mouse proteins or if you have any other allergies, and all OTC and prescription medications you are taking, as well as supplements.
- If you have congestive heart failure, liver disease, a history of cancer, multiple sclerosis, seizures or epilepsy, any current infection or an infection that recurs (e.g., cold sores), a history of hepatitis B or tuberculosis, any condition that affects the blood, certain lung disorders (e.g., chronic obstructive pulmonary disease), and any disease that affects the immune system, including diabetes and HIV/AIDS.

- If you have recently lived or traveled in areas where certain fungal infections (e.g., histoplasmosis, coccidioidomycosis) are common, including the Ohio and Mississippi River valleys and Southwestern United States.
- Before receiving any live vaccines, consult your doctor if you are taking infliximab. This includes the nasal (but not the injected) flu vaccine.

Of Special Interest to Women

- Patients with Crohn's disease or rheumatoid arthritis, especially those who have highly active disease or have been exposed to immunosuppressant therapy, may be at a greater risk for the development of lymphoma or other malignancies.
- It is not known if infliximab passes into breast milk. Therefore, breast-feeding while taking this drug is not recommended.
- Infliximab is a Category B medication, which means it is unlikely to harm the fetus. However, because not all the risks associated with use of the drug are known, you should use infliximab only if your health-care provider deems it is necessary.

Symptoms of Overdose

There have been so few cases of overdose associated with infliximab that the symptoms are not known. If you suspect an overdose, contact your physician immediately.

Letrozole

Brand Name

Femara

Available as Generic?

No

Principal Uses

Breast cancer in postmenopausal women, hormone-sensitive early breast cancer in postmenopausal women after surgery (see "About the Drug")

About the Drug

Letrozole is an antiestrogen drug (nonsteroidal aromatase inhibitor) used to treat breast cancer that depends on the hormone estrogen to grow and spread in postmenopausal women. The drug works by inhibiting the enzyme aromatase in the adrenal glands that produces estrogens, which in turn decreases the amount of estrogen in the body and helps to slow or reverse the growth of breast cancer.

The FDA has approved letrozole as the sole treatment for postmeno-pausal women who have any of the following types of breast cancer:

- Early-stage hormone receptor–positive disease in women who have already tried other treatments
- Early-stage breast cancer that has been treated with tamoxifen for at least 5 years
- Breast cancer that is locally advanced or has spread to other parts of the body (metastasized) and is hormone receptor–positive
- Breast cancer that is locally advanced or has spread and it is not known whether it is hormone receptor–positive or negative
- Advanced breast cancer that has worsened after antiestrogen treatment

How to Use This Drug

Letrozole is available in tablets and is typically taken once daily, with or without food. Take it at the same time each day as directed by your physician.

Side Effects

- Common side effects: chest pain, constipation, diarrhea, dizziness, hair loss, hot flashes, insomnia, joint or bone pain, muscle pain, nausea, tiredness, and unusual sweating.
- Unlikely side effects that should be reported to your doctor: blurry vision, bone fractures, mental/mood changes, and swelling of the arms or legs.
- Rare but very serious side effects that should be reported immediately to your doctor: chest/jaw/left arm pain, confusion, coughing up blood, dark urine, numbness in the legs or arms, slurred speech, sudden shortness of breath, sudden dizziness or fainting, sudden or severe headache, vision changes, weakness on one side of the body, or yellowing of the eyes or skin.

Possible Drug, Supplement, and/or Food Interactions

- Letrozole may reduce the effectiveness of clopidogrel.
- Letrozole with thalidomide increases the risk of thromboembolism. NOTE: Thalidomide is well known for causing birth defects. It is very strictly controlled and only authorized doctors may prescribe it. It is FDA approved for the treatment of Hansen's disease (leprosy), scleroderma, and multiple myeloma (cancer of the white blood cells in bone marrow), and only for women who are postmenopausal.
- Use of any type of estrogen-containing medication should be avoided while taking letrozole because it can negate the effectiveness of letrozole.

Tell Your Doctor
- If you have any allergies and all OTC and prescription medications you are taking, as well as supplements.
- If you have high cholesterol, osteoporosis or osteopenia, stroke, blood clots, heart disease, kidney problems, or liver problems.

Of Special Interest to Women
- Letrozole is usually not prescribed to women of childbearing age. If you are near menopause or have not gone through menopause and your doctor has prescribed letrozole, you should discuss the need for reliable forms of birth control. You should not use birth control products that contain estrogen.
- Letrozole is known to damage a fetus and should not be taken by pregnant women.
- It is not known if letrozole passes into breast milk.
- Letrozole can cause or worsen osteoporosis. Talk to your doctor about what steps you can take to minimize or prevent this occurrence.

Symptoms of Overdose
None expected to cause life-threatening symptoms.

Levonorgestrel Intrauterine System

Brand Name
Mirena

Available as Generic?
No

Principal Use
Prevent pregnancy

About the Drug
Levonorgestrel is a female hormone (progestin) that can cause changes in the cervical mucus and uterine lining, which makes it more difficult for sperm to reach the uterus and for a fertilized egg to attach to the uterine wall. The device does not contain any estrogen. The levonorgestrel intrauterine system consists of a plastic device that contains the hormone. The device is placed in your uterus, where it gradually releases the hormone to prevent pregnancy for up to 5 years.

Levonorgestrel intrauterine device is designed for women who have had at least one child and who are in a stable sexual relationship with a partner who does not have other sexual partners. It can also be used by women who experience heavy menstrual bleeding and who want to use an IUD.

How to Use This Drug

Your physician must insert the levonorgestrel intrauterine system. He or she will use a thin plastic tube to insert the device, which should be put into place within 7 days after the start of your menstrual period. You may experience brief pain, vaginal bleeding, and dizziness while the device is being inserted. These symptoms typically last only about 30 minutes after the device is inserted.

Be sure to follow your doctor's instructions on the care of the device. If for any reason you believe the device has slipped or has shifted, contact your health-care provider as soon as possible. Use a nonhormone method of birth control (e.g., spermicide, condom) until your doctor can replace your IUD.

Do not attempt to remove the device yourself; your health-care provider must do it for you.

Side Effects

- Less serious side effects: back pain, bloating, breakthrough bleeding or heavier menstrual bleeding during the first few weeks of use, breast tenderness or pain, dizziness, headache, irregular menstrual periods, loss of interest in sex, mild itching, mood changes, nausea, nervousness, rash, vomiting, and weight gain.
- Severe pain in your side or lower stomach may be a sign of ectopic pregnancy (development of a fetus in the fallopian tube rather than the uterus), which is a medical emergency. Seek immediate medical attention.
- In rare cases, the device can become embedded in the uterine wall or perforate the uterus. If this occurs, you may experience some of the serious side effects listed below. Your doctor will need to remove the device.
- Serious side effects that require immediate medical attention: easy bleeding or bruising; extreme dizziness; heavy or ongoing vaginal bleeding; pain during intercourse; severe cramps or pelvic pain; severe pain in your side or lower stomach; signs of infection (e.g., fever, chills); sudden numbness or weakness, especially on one side of the body; unusual vaginal discharge; or yellowing of the skin or eyes.

Possible Drug, Supplement, and/or Food Interactions

- Drugs that may affect the effectiveness of the levonorgestrel intrauterine system include insulin, blood thinners (e.g., warfarin), and steroids (e.g., prednisone, fluticasone).
- Griseofulvin and etretinate may interfere with the efficacy of levonorgestrel.

- Levonorgestrel may reduce the concentrations and effects of tizanidine.

Tell Your Doctor

- About any prescription and OTC drugs you are taking, as well as supplements.
- If you are allergic to levonorgestrel, silicone, or polyethylene. You should not use this medication if you have these allergies.
- If you have any of the following conditions, because you should not use this medication if you do: abnormal vaginal bleeding, untreated or uncontrolled vaginal or pelvic infection, a serious pelvic infection following a pregnancy or abortion within the last 3 months, history of pelvic inflammatory disease, uterine fibroid tumors or other conditions that influence the shape of the uterus, history of or current breast cancer, liver disease or tumor, known or suspected cervical or uterine cancer, recent abnormal Pap smear, any condition that weakens your immune system such as leukemia or AIDS.
- If you are currently using an IUD or if your sexual relationship is not exclusive. You should not use this medication.
- If you have diabetes, a bleeding or blood-clotting disorder, a sexually transmitted disease, high blood pressure, heart disease, or a heart valve disorder.

Of Special Interest to Women

- Contact your doctor immediately if you become pregnant while using the levonorgestrel intrauterine system. You may experience a severe infection, miscarriage, premature birth, or death.
- If you are breast-feeding, wait at least 6 weeks before you begin using the levonorgestrel intrauterine system.
- You may experience irregular periods during the first 3–6 months after the device has been inserted.
- If you have more than one sexual partner, or your partner has sexual partners besides you, do not use the levonorgestrel intrauterine system. This device may increase your risk of developing a serious pelvic infection.
- Contact your doctor immediately if your sexual partner develops any sexually transmitted disease. Remember, use of levonorgestrel intrauterine system does not protect you against STDs.

Symptoms of Overdose

Overdose is highly unlikely.

Levothyroxine

Brand Names

Levothroid, Levoxyl, Synthroid, Unithroid

Available as Generic?

Yes. However, that generic and branded tablets of levothyroxine may differ in the amount of drug they contain, the rate of absorption of the drug into the body, and the distribution of the drug throughout the body.

Principal Uses

Hypothyroidism, suppression of thyroid hormone release to manage cancerous thyroid nodules and the growth of goiters, manage thyrotoxicosis

About the Drug

Levothyroxine is a synthetic version of thyroxine (T-4), the main thyroid hormone produced and released by the thyroid gland. It is prescribed for individuals whose thyroid gland is not producing enough of the hormone. The goal of treatment with levothyroxine is to achieve and maintain a normal blood thyroxine level. This hormone plays a major role in the growth and development of bone, the brain, and other tissues in the body. Thyroid hormone helps to maintain brain function, metabolism, and body temperature, among other activities.

Because different brands and generics of levothyroxine may not work the same way, you should keep taking the same brand or generic to avoid fluctuations.

How to Use This Drug

Levothyroxine is available in tablets and as a dry powder (for intravenous use in a hospital or other health facility). Always take the tablets with 8 ounces of water because they can dissolve rapidly and swell in your throat. Take levothyroxine on an empty stomach, 30 minutes before eating.

The typical starting dose for hypothyroidism is 12.5–125 mcg per day. Your physician will determine your dose based on your age, the presence of other medical conditions, blood levels of thyroid hormone, and other factors. It may take 1–3 weeks after starting treatment before you notice the effects of the drug.

Side Effects

- Most people tolerate levothyroxine very well. Any side effects are usually related to toxic levels of thyroid hormone and are symptoms of hyperthyroidism. These may include chest pain, diarrhea, excessive sweating, fever, headache, heat intolerance, increased heart rate or pulse, insomnia, irregular menstrual cycles, nervousness, vomiting, and weight loss.

- Rarely, some hair loss occurs during the first few months of starting levothyroxine. This is temporary in most cases. If it persists, contact your doctor.
- Rarely, serious side effects occur, including chest pain, rapid or irregular heartbeat, shortness of breath, and seizures.

Possible Drug, Supplement, and/or Food Interactions

- You may experience irregular heart rhythm if you use antidepressants along with levothyroxine.
- Foods that are high in fiber—e.g., peas, beans, lentils, artichoke, raspberries—may decrease your body's ability to absorb levothyroxine.
- The following medications can be taken along with levothyroxine but they may make levothryoxine less effective: antacids that contain aluminum, calcium carbonate, cholesterol-lowering drugs (e.g., cholestyramine, colestipol), ferrous sulfate iron supplements, sucralfate, and sodium polystyrene sulfonate. Use them at least 4 hours before or after you take levothyroxine.
- If you take insulin or antidiabetic drugs, starting or discontinuing levothyroxine may result in your need to change your dose of diabetic medication.
- Levothyroxine may increase the effect of blood thinners such as warfarin.
- Use of intravenous epinephrine by patients who have coronary artery disease and who are using levothyroxine may cause breathing difficulties and heart attack.
- Levothyroxine may reduce the effectiveness of some beta-blocking drugs (e.g., metoprolol, propranolol) and of digoxin.
- Do not use any type of diet pills while taking levothyroxine because you may experience serious, even life-threatening, effects.

Tell Your Doctor

- If you have any allergies and all prescription and OTC medications you are taking, as well as supplements.
- If you have recently undergone radiation treatment with iodine.
- If you have adrenal gland problems, anemia, coronary artery disease, diabetes, heart disease, history of blood clots, or pituitary gland problems.

- If you have had a heart attack, a thyroid disease called thyrotoxicosis, or an uncontrollable adrenal gland condition. You should not take levothyroxine if you have any of these issues.

Of Special Interest to Women

- Levothyroxine is a pregnancy category A drug, which means it is safe to use while you are pregnant and breast-feeding. Even though the drug passes into breast milk, it is not expected to cause harm to a nursing infant.
- Tell your doctor if you become pregnant or you begin breast-feeding during treatment, because he or she may need to increase your dose.
- In most cases, levothyroxine must be taken for the rest of a person's life. Because prolonged use of levothyroxine can cause bone loss and result in osteoporosis, talk to your health-care provider about the steps you need to take to avoid osteoporosis.

Symptoms of Overdose

Chest pain, confusion, diarrhea, pounding heartbeat, leg cramps, seizures, shortness of breath, and vomiting.

Lisinopril

Brand Names

Prinivil, Zestril

Available as Generic?

Yes

Principal Uses

High blood pressure, heart failure, improve survival following a heart attack

About the Drug

Lisinopril is an angiotensin-converting enzyme ACE inhibitor. Other drugs in this category include captopril (Capoten), enalapril (Vasotec), quinapril (Accupril), and ramipril (Altace). Angiotensin is a chemical produced by the body that causes the blood vessels to narrow, which results in a rise in blood pressure. Lisinopril blocks the enzyme that converts angiotensin into its active form, which allows the blood vessels to dilate and blood pressure to fall.

How to Use This Drug

Lisinopril is available in tablets and can be taken with or without food. Take lisinopril at the same time each day for best results. The starting dose is usually 5 mg daily, and the effective dose range for people who have heart failure is 5–40 mg daily. Doses can be increased by 10 mg every 2 weeks by your physician. The maximum dose is 40 mg daily. It may take several weeks or months before you get the full benefit from lisinopril for congestive heart failure.

The usual starting dose for high blood pressure is 10 mg daily, with the usual range 20–40 mg daily. Higher doses are not better, so 40 mg provide about the same effect as do 80 mg.

For treatment of heart attack, the typical starting dose is 5 mg followed by 5 mg after 24 hours, 10 mg after 48 hours, and then 10 mg daily. Generally you will need to take lisinopril for 6 weeks following a heart attack.

Side Effects

- Most common side effects: anxiety, blurry vision, dizziness (the first doses of lisinopril can cause dizziness because of a drop in blood pressure), drowsiness, dry cough, fatigue, insomnia, nasal congestion, and nausea.
- Unlikely but serious side effects: change in the amount of urine, chest pain, decreased sexual drive, fainting, signs of infection (e.g., chills, fever, persistent sore throat), or vision changes.
- Rarely, lisinopril causes a decline in the levels of red blood cells, white blood cells, and platelets.
- Lisinopril rarely causes serious and possibly fatal liver problems. Warning signs and symptoms include abdominal pain, dark urine, persistent fatigue, persistent nausea, and yellowing of the skin or eyes.

Possible Drug, Supplement, and/or Food Interactions

- Lisinopril with potassium supplements or diuretics that conserve potassium (e.g., hydrochlorothiazide/triamterene) may cause your blood potassium levels to rise to a dangerous level.
- Injectable gold (used to treat rheumatoid arthritis) with lisinopril may cause nitritoid reactions, with symptoms of facial flushing, nausea, vomiting, and low blood pressure.
- Lisinopril may interact negatively with NSAIDs, such as celecoxib, ibuprofen, indomethacin; lithium; trimethoprim-containing medications (e.g., sulfamethoxazole/trimethoprim); and drugs that suppress the immune system (e.g., azathioprine).

Tell Your Doctor

- If you have any allergies, especially to other ACE inhibitors, as well as to bee or wasp stings, and also all OTC and prescription medications you are taking, as well as supplements.

- If you have kidney problems, as lisinopril can impair kidney function.
- If you have a history of allergic reactions (e.g., swelling of the face, lips, tongue, throat), kidney disease, liver disease, high blood levels of potassium, severe dehydration, blood vessel disease (e.g., lupus, scleroderma).

Of Special Interest to Women
- Fetuses and newborns have died when women took lisinopril during pregnancy.
- It is not known whether lisinopril passes into breast milk. Discuss breast-feeding with your physician.

Symptoms of Overdose
Fainting, severe dizziness, and unusually fast or slow heartbeat.

Lubiprostone

Brand Name
Amitiza

Available as Generic?
No

Principal Uses
Idiopathic (unknown cause) chronic constipation, irritable bowel syndrome with constipation

About the Drug
Lubiprostone was approved by the FDA in 2006 for treatment of chronic constipation of unknown cause, and for treatment of irritable bowel syndrome with constipation in 2008. Lubiprostone causes an increase in the secretion of fluid into the intestinal tract, which softens stool and facilitates its movement through the intestinal tract, and can also relieve the pain and discomfort associated with chronic constipation.

How to Use This Drug
Lubiprostone is available in capsules and can be taken with food. Take lubiprostone with a full glass of water. Usual dosing is 24 mcg twice daily. Do not break or chew the capsules.

Side Effects
- Most common side effects: diarrhea and nausea.
- Less common side effects: anxiety; bloating; decreased appetite; dizziness; fecal incontinence; frequent bowel movements; headache; joint or muscle pain; rash; stomach pain; and swelling in the hands, feet, or ankles.

- Within 1 hour of taking lubiprostone, some people experience tightness in the chest or shortness of breath. These side effects typically disappear within 3 hours, but they recur when you take your next dose. Tell your doctor if these side effects become bothersome.

Possible Drug, Supplement, and/or Food Interactions

No drug, supplement, or food interactions have been reported thus far. However, this does not mean interactions are not possible. Report any unusual symptoms to your health-care provider.

Tell Your Doctor

- If you have any allergies, and all prescription and OTC medications, as well as supplements, you are taking.
- If you have a history of hernia, gallstones, Crohn's disease, Hirschsprung's disease, diverticulitis, polyps, or any other cause of obstruction of the gastrointestinal tract.
- If you are pregnant or become pregnant during treatment.

Of Special Interest to Women

- Taking lubiprostone during pregnancy has not been studied adequately. Discuss the benefits and risks associated with use of this drug with your physician.
- It is not known whether lubiprostone passes into breast milk. If you are breast-feeding, do not take this medication without telling your doctor.

Symptoms of Overdose

Not known, but they likely would include more serious levels of the common side effects, including nausea, diarrhea, and vomiting.

Mefenamic Acid

Brand Name

Ponstel

Available as Generic?

Yes

Principal Uses

Short-term relief from mild to moderate pain; to reduce pain and blood loss from menstrual periods

About the Drug

Mefenamic acid is an NSAID that works by reducing the levels of hormones (prostaglandins) that cause inflammation, fever, and pain. It can be taken for a wide range of painful conditions, but it should not be taken for the treatment of peri-operative pain if you are undergoing coronary artery bypass graft surgery.

How to Use This Drug

Mefenamic acid is available in capsules and should be taken with a full glass of water, typically 4 times daily. If you experience stomach upset, take the medication with food. Do not lie down for at least 30 minutes after taking mefenamic acid. Do not take mefenamic acid for more than 7 days at a time without consulting your health-care provider.

If you are using mefenamic acid on an as-needed basis, take it at the first sign of pain, as this medication is less effective if you wait until your pain has worsened. For menstrual pain, take your first dose as soon as your period begins.

Side Effects

- Common side effects: diarrhea, dizziness, drowsiness, headache, heartburn, nausea, and upset stomach.
- Unlikely but serious side effects that should be reported to your health-care provider immediately: change in the color or amount of urine; difficult or painful swallowing; easy bruising or bleeding; fainting; hearing changes; mental/mood changes; rapidly pounding heartbeat; stomach pain; swelling of the ankles, feet, or hands; unexplained stiff neck.
- Rare but very serious side effects that require immediate medical attention: black stools, chest pain, persistent nausea/vomiting, vomit that looks like coffee grounds, severe dizziness, slurred speech, trouble breathing, weakness on one side of the body, and yellowing of the skin or eyes.
- Mefenamic acid and other NSAIDs may increase the risk of life-threatening cardiovascular thrombotic events, heart attack, and stroke. This risk may increase the longer you take the medication, and is greater among individuals who have cardiovascular disease or risk factors for cardiovascular disease.

Possible Drug, Supplement, and/or Food Interactions

- Certain antacids can change the amount of mefenamic acid your body absorbs.
- Mefenamic with cidofovir or ketorolac can result in very serious interactions.
- Mefenamic may interact with certain herbs and supplements to increase the risk of bleeding: dong quai, feverfew, fish oil supplements, garlic, ginger, ginkgo biloba, ginseng, Saint-John's-wort.

- Blood pressure medications such as ACE inhibitors (e.g., captopril), angiotensin II receptor blockers (losartan), or beta-blockers (e.g., metoprolol) with mefenamic acid may reduce the blood pressure–lowering effects of the blood pressure drugs.
- Mefenamic acid with NSAIDs (e.g., aspirin, ibuprofen) or corticosteroids can increase the risk of bleeding. Consult your health-care provider if you are taking aspirin to help prevent heart attack or stroke.
- Mefenamic acid may reduce the effectiveness of diuretics (e.g., furosemide, hydrochlorothiazide).
- Mefenamic acid with lithium may increase the amount of lithium in your body.
- Mefenamic acid with methotrexate should be monitored by your health-care provider.
- Mefenamic acid with cyclosporine may increase your risk of kidney damage.
- Mefenamic acid may interfere with the results of certain lab tests. Tell your physician and lab personnel if you are taking this medication.
- Alcohol with mefenamic acid may increase your risk of stomach bleeding.
- Mefenamic acid may make you more sensitive to sunlight. Avoid prolonged exposure to the sun, tanning booths, and sunlamps.

Tell Your Doctor
- If you have any allergies and all OTC and prescription medications you are taking, as well as supplements.
- If you have asthma (especially aspirin-sensitive asthma); kidney disease; recent heart bypass surgery; active gastrointestinal bleeding or ulcers; blood disorders; high blood pressure dehydration; diabetes; heart disease; liver disease; nasal polyps; obesity; history of gastrointestinal problems; stroke; swelling of the ankles, feet, and/or hands.

Of Special Interest to Women
- If used during pregnancy, mefenamic acid should be taken only during the first 6 months if your health-care provider believes it is necessary. It is not recommended during the last trimester because it may harm the fetus and/or interfere with normal labor and delivery.
- Mefenamic acid passes into breast milk. Consult your health-care provider about breast-feeding.

Symptoms of Overdose

Extreme drowsiness, seizures, severe stomach pain, slowed breathing, and vomit that looks like coffee grounds.

Metformin

Brand Names

Fortamet, Glucophage, Glucophage XR, Glumetza, Riomet

Available as Generic?

Yes

Principal Uses

Type 2 diabetes, polycystic ovarian syndrome

About the Drug

Metformin is an oral antidiabetes medication that belongs to the class of drugs called biguanides. Metformin works by increasing sensitivity of the liver, fat, muscles, and other tissues to the uptake and effects of insulin and lowering the level of glucose (sugar) in the bloodstream. Insulin is a hormone produced by the pancreas that controls the amount of glucose in your blood in two ways: by reducing how much glucose the liver makes, and by increasing the amount of glucose that is removed from the blood by fat and muscle. When these activities work properly, blood glucose levels fall.

If you have type 2 diabetes, your body has an insufficient amount of insulin. Metformin increases your body's ability to utilize the insulin you have, which in turn lowers your glucose levels.

Studies show that metformin can reduce the complications of diabetes, such as blindness, kidney disease, heart disease, and neuropathy. Unlike the glucose-lowering drugs used to treat type 2 diabetes (e.g., glyburide, glipizide), metformin does not lower the concentration of insulin in the blood and therefore does not cause abnormally low blood glucose levels (hypoglycemia). Metformin may be used alone or along with other diabetic medications.

How to Use This Drug

Metformin is available in regular and extended-release tablets. It is usually taken with meals, and you should drink plenty of fluids while taking this medication unless your doctor gives you other directions. The regular tablets are usually taken 2–3 times daily, while the extended-release may be taken once or twice daily. It may take up to 2 weeks before metformin is effective, and your doctor may need to adjust your dose based on your blood sugar levels. The usual maximum dose is 2000 mg of the regular tablets and 2550 mg daily of the extended-release, or as directed by your doctor.

Metformin works best if you also eat a healthful diet and get regular moderate exercise to control blood sugar levels. This combination of medication and lifestyle changes can help prevent the complications associated with type 2 diabetes.

If you have polycystic ovarian syndrome, your doctor may prescribe metformin to help your body better respond to insulin. Better response to insulin can help reduce your risk of diabetes, regulate your menstrual cycle, and improve fertility.

Side Effects

- Common side effects: bloating, diarrhea, gas, loss of appetite, nausea, and vomiting. Approximately one-third of patients experience these symptoms, and they can be severe enough to cause about 5% of individuals to stop taking the medication. Side effects can be lessened if the dose is reduced.
- A serious but rare side effect is lactic acidosis, which occurs in 1 out of every 30,000 users and is fatal in 50% of cases. Symptoms include abnormal heartbeat, breathing difficulties, feeling cold, light-headedness, stomach discomfort, and unusual muscle pain.
- Metformin usually does not cause hypoglycemia (abnormally low blood sugar), but it may occur if you are taking other medications for diabetes, drink large amounts of alcohol, perform vigorous exercise, or do not eat enough calories from food. Symptoms include blurry vision, cold sweats, dizziness, drowsiness, fainting, fast heartbeat, headache, hunger, shaking, and tingling of the hands or feet.

Possible Drug, Supplement, and/or Food Interactions

- Cimetidine, cephalexin, furosemide, and thiazide diuretics affect the kidneys' ability to eliminate metformin from the body. Cimetidine especially can increase the amount of metformin in the blood by 40%.
- Beta-blockers (e.g., propranolol) may cover up symptoms of hypoglycemia, such as pounding or rapid heartbeat.
- Check the labels on all prescription and OTC drugs as well as supplements to see if they contain sugar or alcohol, as these ingredients may affect your blood sugar levels.

Tell Your Doctor
- If you have any allergies and all prescription and OTC medications you take, as well as supplements.
- Before you start, stop, or change any medication, talk to your doctor about how the medication may affect your blood sugar levels.
- If you have kidney disease, liver disease, metabolic acidosis, any type of serious infection, dehydration, or any condition that can cause a low level of oxygen in the blood or poor circulation (e.g., recent heart attack or stroke).
- If you have a history of severe breathing problems, adrenal or pituitary gland conditions, blood problems, fertility difficulties, or alcohol use.
- Before you have surgery or any type of scanning procedure that uses injectable iodinated contrast materials, tell your doctor that you are taking metformin. You will need to stop taking metformin temporarily before these procedures.

Of Special Interest to Women
- No adequate studies of metformin in pregnant women have been conducted. Experts generally agree that insulin is the best treatment for type 2 diabetes in pregnant women.
- Metformin is excreted into breast milk, so you should not breast-feed.
- Metformin can change your menstrual cycle and promote ovulation, which increases the risk of becoming pregnant.

Symptoms of Overdose
Rapid breathing, slow or irregular heartbeat, and severe drowsiness.

Methotrexate

Brand Names
Rheumatrex, Trexall
Available as Generic?
Yes
Principal Uses
Cancer, rheumatoid arthritis, psoriasis, psoriatic arthritis, polymyositis, lupus
About the Drug
Methotrexate is an antimetabolite, which means it blocks the metabolism of cells. Because of this, methotrexate can be effective in treating

diseases that involve abnormally rapid cell growth, such as cancer and psoriasis. Methotrexate is also helpful in the treatment of rheumatic diseases, including rheumatoid arthritis, although exactly how it works in these conditions is not known.

How to Use This Drug

Methotrexate is available in tablets and as an injection and can be taken with or without food. The dosing schedules for methotrexate vary greatly, especially if you are taking it for cancer, so be sure you follow your doctor's directions carefully. For rheumatoid arthritis or psoriasis, you will likely take the drug once a week by injection or orally. It can take several months of continued use before you experience the full benefits of methotrexate. Drink lots of fluids while taking methotrexate to help your kidneys remove the drug from your body and minimize some of its side effects.

Side Effects

- Common side effects: dizziness, drowsiness, headache, low white blood counts, mouth sores, nausea, stomach pain, and vomiting.
- Severe toxicity of the liver, kidneys, and bone marrow can occur with methotrexate.
- Serious side effects that should be reported to your doctor immediately: black stools, bone pain, dark urine, diarrhea, enlarged glands or lymph nodes, persistent sore throat, unusual bleeding or bruising, and unusual pain or skin discoloration.
- A dry nonproductive cough may indicate a rare lung toxicity. Report it to your physician.
- Highly unlikely but serious side effects that you should report immediately: breathing difficulties, calf pain or swelling, chest pain, irregular heartbeat, mental/mood changes, muscle weakness, vision changes, and yellowing of the skin or eyes.
- Very infrequently, abnormal growths or tumors may appear while taking methotrexate. Contact your health-care provider immediately.
- On rare occasions, methotrexate with radiation may increase the risk of tissue and bone damage.

Possible Drug, Supplement, and/or Food Interactions

- Methotrexate with any of the following drugs may result in very serious interactions: acitretin, asparaginase, live vaccines (e.g., BCG for tuberculosis, nasal seasonal flu), natalizumab, and pyrimethamine.

- The following drugs may also interact with methotrexate: other cancer treatments (e.g., cisplatin), ciprofloxacin, digoxin, leflunomide, drugs toxic to the liver (e.g., azathioprine, sulfasalazine), penicillins, phenytoin, probenecid, procarbazine, sulfa drugs, theophylline.
- Some antibiotics (e.g., chloramphenicol, sulfa, tetracyclines) may interfere with blood tests for methotrexate. Tell lab personnel and your health-care provider if you are using antibiotics.
- Methotrexate (usually high doses) with NSAIDs (e.g., indomethacin, ketoprofen) can, rarely, cause severe or fatal bone marrow suppression and gastrointestinal bleeding.
- NSAIDs, including low-dose aspirin for prevention of stroke and heart attack, with low-dose methotrexate should be closely monitored by your health-care provider.

Tell Your Doctor
- If you use alcohol, have blood cell or bone marrow disorders, liver disease, severe kidney disease, severe lung disease, or a suppressed immune system. You should not use methotrexate.
- If you have a history of intestinal or stomach disease (e.g., peptic ulcer, ulcerative colitis), kidney disease, an active infection, or a folic acid deficiency.

Of Special Interest to Women
- Do not use methotrexate if you are pregnant or plan to get pregnant, as this drug can be toxic to the fetus and cause birth defects and miscarriage. Discontinue use of methotrexate for at least one ovulatory cycle before conception. Male partners should stop using methotrexate at least 3 months before a planned conception. If you become pregnant while taking methotrexate, contact your doctor immediately.
- Methotrexate is excreted in breast milk and should not be used if you are breast-feeding.
- Methotrexate can make you hypersensitive to the sun, so avoid prolonged exposure to sunlight, tanning booths, and sunlamps.

Symptoms of Overdose
Bloody stools, severe nausea, and severe vomiting.

Methylprednisolone

Brand Names
Medrol, Medrol Dosepak

Available as Generic?

Yes

Principal Uses

Inflammatory conditions, including but not limited to rheumatoid arthritis, lupus, acute gouty arthritis, psoriatic arthritis, ulcerative colitis, and Crohn's disease; also severe allergic conditions that do not respond to conventional treatment, such as allergic rhinitis and bronchial asthma; chronic skin conditions such as severe psoriasis

About the Drug

Methylprednisolone is a synthetic corticosteroid (steroid). Corticosteroids are naturally produced by the body and have varying effects on metabolism and the immune system, and also block inflammation. Methylprednisolone prevents the release of substances in the body that cause inflammation.

How to Use This Drug

Methylprednisolone is available in tablets and as an injection. Take the tablets with food or milk and a full glass of water. If you are taking the tablets, the initial dose is 4–48 mg daily. If you are using an injection, how you inject the medication—into a vein or muscle—will depend on the brand and strength your doctor has prescribed.

Whenever possible, the lowest effective dose is taken for the shortest length of time to minimize side effects. Your doctor may prescribe every-other-day dosing to help reduce side effects. If you take methylpredisolone once daily, it is recommended you take it before 9 A.M.

Prolonged use of methylprednisolone can suppress the ability of your adrenal glands to produce corticosteroids. Therefore, do not suddenly stop taking methylprednisolone, because it can cause corticosteroid insufficiency, which can cause nausea, vomiting, extreme fatigue, and even shock. Consult your health-care provider about how to taper off this drug.

Side Effects

- Common side effects: dizziness, fluid retention, headache, increased appetite, menstrual period changes, pain/redness/swelling at the injection site, sleep problems, stomach upset, and weight gain.
- Less likely but serious side effects: cataracts, glaucoma, convulsions, depression, euphoria, hair growth on the face, high blood pressure, insomnia, mood swings, muscle weakness, potassium loss, puffiness of the face, and thinning and easy bruising of the skin.
- Unlikely but serious side effects that should be reported immediately to your health-care provider: bone or joint pain, easy bruising or bleed-

ing, black stools, fast/irregular heartbeat, increased thirst or urination, muscle weakness or pain, seizures, shortness of breath, swollen ankles or feet, unusual skin growths, vision changes, and vomit that looks like coffee grounds.

Possible Drug, Supplement, and/or Food Interactions

- Do not get any live vaccines while taking methylprednisolone because the combination may lead to very serious interactions.
- Methylprednisolone may interfere with the results of certain lab tests, including skin tests. Tell your doctor and lab personnel you are using this drug.
- Clarithyromycin, erythromycin, and ketoconazole can reduce the liver's ability to metabolize methylprednisolone, resulting in higher blood levels of the drug and a greater risk of side effects.
- Birth control pills and estrogens can increase the effect of methylprednisolone by 50%.
- Cyclosporine reduces the metabolism of methylprednisolone, and methylprednisolone reduces the metabolism of cyclosporine.
- Methylprednisolone may decrease or increase the effect of blood thinners (e.g., warfarin).
- Phenobarbital, phenytoin, and rifampin may increase the metabolism of methylprednisolone and thus reduce its effectiveness.
- The following drugs and herbs may interact with methylprednisolone: aldesleukin, bupropion, diabetes medications, licorice, mifepristone, and natalizumab.
- Aspirin, salicylates, and NSAIDs (e.g., ibuprofen) may increase the risk of stomach bleeding.
- Avoid contact with anyone who has recently had a polio vaccine. Seek immediate medical attention if you come into contact with anyone who has chicken pox or measles.
- Methylprednisolone may change your blood sugar levels, so if you use diabetes medications, your dosing may need to be modified.
- Alcohol may increase the risk of gastrointestinal bleeding.

Tell Your Doctor

- If you have any allergies and all OTC and prescription medications you are taking, as well as supplements.
- If you have any untreated, active fungal infections, because you should not take methylprednisolone.
- If you have bleeding problems, a history of blood clots, osteoporosis, high blood pressure, heart problems, diabetes, cataracts, glaucoma,

herpes infection, kidney disease, a current infection (e.g., tuberculosis), severe liver disease, mental/mood conditions (e.g., psychosis, depression), seizures, gastrointestinal problems (e.g., ulcer, ulcerative colitis), hypothyroidism, or untreated mineral problems (e.g., low potassium or calcium).

- If you plan to have surgery, including dental surgery, tell your doctor or dentist that you are taking methylprednisolone or if you have used it within the last year.

Of Special Interest to Women

- Methylprednisolone should be used during pregnancy only if your health-care provider decides it is necessary. In rare cases, infants born to women who took methylprednisolone for a long time had low levels of corticosteroid hormone, which can cause persistent nausea/vomiting, severe diarrhea, and weakness.
- Methylprednisolone passes into breast milk. Although there are no reports of harm to nursing infants, discuss the benefits and risks of breast-feeding with your health-care provider.
- Methylprednisolone hinders the absorption of calcium and contributes to the development of osteoporosis. Calcium and vitamin D supplements are recommended to slow or stop bone loss.

Symptoms of Overdose

An overdose of methylprednisolone is not expected to be life-threatening. Long-term use of high doses may cause acne, changes in the location or shape of body fat (especially in the face, neck, and waist), easy bruising, loss of libido, menstrual problems, and thinning skin.

Metoprolol

Brand Names

Lopressor, Toprol XL

Available as Generic?

Yes

Principal Uses

High blood pressure, chest pain (angina pectoris) related to coronary artery disease, prevention of migraine

About the Drug

Metoprolol is a beta-adrenergic blocking agent, a drug class that also includes atenolol (Tenormin), propanolol (Inderal), and timolol (Blocadren). Metoprolol interferes with the activity of the sympathetic nervous system by blocking beta receptors on sympathetic nerves. Because the sympathetic nervous system is responsible for increased heart rate, blocking the action of these nerves reduces heart rate and is thus helpful in treating abnormally rapid heart rhythms.

Metoprolol lowers blood pressure by reducing the force of the contractions of the heart muscle. When heart rate and muscle contractions are reduced, the heart muscle needs less oxygen. By reducing the heart's demand for oxygen, metoprolol is effective in treating heart pain (angina).

How to Use This Drug

Metoprolol is available as traditional and extended-release tablets, as well as via injection. Generally metoprolol is taken before meals or at bedtime. For high blood pressure, a typical dose is 100–450 mg daily in 1 or divided doses. For angina, a usual dose is 100–400 mg daily in 2 divided doses. For acute myocardial infarction (heart attack), you will likely receive 3 injections given 2 minutes apart, followed by oral metoprolol for at least 3 months. It can take 1 or 2 weeks before the full benefits of metoprolol take effect.

If you have angina or heart disease, do not suddenly stop taking metoprolol. Your doctor will help you gradually reduce your dose. When gradually stopping metoprolol, seek immediate medical attention if you develop worsening chest pain and/or chest pain that spreads to other parts of the body, difficulty breathing, sweating, or pressure in the chest.

If you have diabetes, metoprolol can cover up early warning symptoms of low blood sugar, so use this drug with caution. If you have a slow heart rate or heart block, metoprolol may cause your heart rate to become dangerously slow and may even cause shock.

Side Effects

- Common side effects: abdominal cramps, cold extremities (which can be worsened by smoking), constipation, depression, diarrhea, vivid dreams, fatigue, fever, insomnia, light-headedness, low blood pressure, memory loss, shortness of breath, sore throat, vision changes, and wheezing.
- Metoprolol may worsen breathing problems if you have asthma, chronic bronchitis, or emphysema.
- Unlikely but serious side effects that you should report immediately to your doctor: bluish discoloration of the fingers or toes, breathing difficulties, cough, increased urination, dark urine, easy bruising or bleeding, fainting, increased thirst, mental/mood changes, numbness

or tingling in the hands or feet, persistent fever or sore throat, persistent nausea, sudden weight gain, and yellowing of the skin or eyes.

Possible Drug, Supplement, and/or Food Interactions
- Calcium channel blockers (e.g., diltiazem, verapamil) and digoxin (Lanoxin) can significantly lower blood pressure and heart rate if you take them with metoprolol. The effects can be life-threatening in some cases.
- Aminophylline, theophylline, and other bronchodilators may cause severe, even fatal, bronchospasms if taken with metoprolol.
- Other drugs that may cause adverse reactions if taken with metoprolol include amiodarone, certain antidepressants (e.g., bupropion, fluoxetine), antidiabetic drugs (e.g., glipizide), barbiturates, cimetidine, epinephrine, NSAIDs, quinidine, rifampin, ritonavir, and the herb Saint-John's-wort.

Tell Your Doctor
- If you have any allergies, including allergies to other beta-blockers.
- All OTC and prescription medications you are taking, as well as supplements.
- If you have blood circulation problems, breathing problems (e.g., asthma), cardiogenic shock, certain types of irregular heartbeat (e.g., sinus bradycardia), diabetes, hyperthyroidism, liver disease, mental/mood disorders, myasthenia gravis, severe heart failure, skin conditions (e.g., psoriasis), or a tumor of the adrenal gland (pheochromocytoma).

Of Special Interest to Women
- Experts have not determined whether metoprolol is safe to take during pregnancy. Consult your health-care provider about the benefits and risks.
- Metoprolol passes into breast milk and may cause adverse effects in infants.

Symptoms of Overdose
Abnormally slow heartbeat, fainting, severe dizziness, slow or shallow breathing, and weakness.

Milnacipran

Brand Name
Savella

Available as Generic?
No

Principal Use

Fibromyalgia

About the Drug

Milnacipran is a selective serotonin and norepinephrine reuptake inhibitor, a class that includes desvenlafaxine (Pristiq), duloxetine (Cymbalta), and venlafaxine (Effexor). Although SNRIs are typically prescribed for depression, milnacipran was approved by the FDA in 2009 as a treatment for fibromyalgia. SNRIs work by preventing the reuptake of serotonin and norepinephrine by nerves after they have been released in the brain. This increases the impact of these neurotransmitters in the brain, and in patients with fibromyalgia it helps stop the transmission of pain signals.

How to Use This Drug

Milnacipran is available in tablets and is usually taken twice daily. You can take milnacipran with or without food, but taking it with food reduces your chances of an upset stomach. Your doctor may start you on a low dose and gradually increase it until you reach an effective level. The typical dose is 50 mg twice daily, with a maximum of 100 mg twice daily. Some women experience relief as quickly as 1 week after starting treatment.

Do not suddenly stop taking milnacipran, which may cause you to experience withdrawal symptoms, such as agitation, dizziness, irritability, mood changes, ringing in your ears, seizures, or tingling/numbness in your hands or feet. Talk to your doctor about tapering off.

Side Effects

- Most frequent side effects: constipation (16% of patients), dizziness (10%), dry mouth, excessive sweating, flushing, headache (18%), high blood pressure, increased heart rate, insomnia, nausea (more than 33%), palpitations, and vomiting.
- Less likely but serious side effects that should be reported to your health-care provider immediately: black/tarry or bloody stools, breathing difficulties, confusion, difficulty concentrating, fainting, fast or pounding heartbeat, hallucinations, lack of energy, loss of appetite, memory problems, nosebleeds, pain in the upper right side of the stomach, seizures, unsteady gait, unusual bleeding or bruising, weakness, vomit that looks like coffee grounds or contains blood.
- Milnacipran with other antidepressants may increase the risk of suicidal thinking and behavior in young people up to about age 24.

Possible Drug, Supplement, and/or Food Interactions

- Do not use milnacipran with MAOIs such as phenelzine, tranylcypromine, and selegiline, or within 14 days of discontinuing an MAOI.

Combining SNRIs and MAOIs may result in serious, sometimes fatal, reactions. Similar reactions may occur if milnacipran is used with antipsychotics, tricyclic antidepressants, and other drugs that impact serotonin levels, such as tryptophan and sumatriptan.

- Milnacipran with epinephrine or norepinephrine may result in high blood pressure and abnormal heartbeats.
- Milnacipran with aspirin and other NSAIDs, warfarin, or other drugs associated with bleeding may increase the risk of bleeding.
- Drinking alcohol while taking milnacipran may increase the risk of liver damage.
- Medications to treat colds or allergies, narcotic pain medicines, sleeping pills, muscle relaxants, and medications for seizures, depression, or anxiety can increase the drowsiness caused by milnacipran.

Tell Your Doctor
- About any allergies you have, including allergies to aspirin, other medications, or tartrazine (FD&C yellow no. 5).
- If you are taking any prescription and OTC medications, as well as supplements, especially 5-HTP or tryptophan.
- If you have ever had an alcohol problem; high blood pressure; seizure or epilepsy; a bleeding or blood-clotting disorder; irregular heartbeat; glaucoma; difficulty urinating; or heart, kidney, or liver disease.
- If you plan to have surgery, including dental surgery, tell your surgeon or dentist you are taking milnacipran.

Of Special Interest to Women
- There are no adequate studies in pregnant women regarding milnacipran. Discuss the benefits and risks with your health-care provider.
- It is not known whether milnacipran passes into breast milk. Use of milnacipran while breast-feeding is not recommended.

Symptoms of Overdose
Coma, confusion, dizziness, extreme sleepiness, and slowed or stopped breathing or heartbeat.

Montelukast

Brand Name
Singulair

Available as Generic?
Yes

Principal Uses

Asthma, seasonal allergic rhinitis (hay fever, ragweed allergy)

About the Drug

Montelukast is a leukotriene receptor antagonist. Leukotrienes are chemicals that occur naturally in the body and promote inflammation in asthma and seasonal allergic rhinitis and other conditions in which inflammation plays a part. When leukotrienes bind to other cells, they stimulate the cells to promote inflammation. Montelukast works by blocking some leukotrienes from binding to other cells, thus reducing inflammation and symptoms related to asthma and seasonal allergic rhinitis, including sneezing, stuffy and/or runny nose, and breathing difficulties.

How to Use This Drug

Montelukast is available in regular and chewable tablets and granules, which can be mixed with food. It begins to relieve symptoms 3–14 days after starting treatment. The recommended dose of montelukast is 4, 5, or 10 mg daily. For asthma, the dose should be taken in the evening with or without food. If you need montelukast to prevent exercise-induced asthma, take your dose 2 hours before exercise. For allergy symptoms, it can be taken anytime of the day.

Montelukast should not be used to treat a sudden attack of asthma symptoms. Your doctor can prescribe a short-acting inhaler for such attacks.

Side Effects

- Common side effects: dizziness, headache, heartburn, inflamed lining of the nose, sore throat, stomach pain, and tiredness. Between 2% and 12% of patients experience these side effects.
- Less common and sometimes serious side effects: breathing difficulties; fever; flulike symptoms; hoarseness; itching; nosebleed; pins and needles or numbness in the arms or legs; rash; swollen sinuses; swollen face, throat, tongue, lips, eyes, hands, feet, ankles, or lower legs.
- Montelukast can have a negative impact on mental health. If you experience any of the following symptoms while taking the drug, contact your doctor immediately: agitation, aggressive behavior, anxiety, depression, hallucinations, irritability, restlessness, sleepwalking or sleep difficulties, suicidal thoughts or actions, or tremors.

Possible Drug, Supplement, and/or Food Interactions

- Phenobarbital or rifampin increases the blood concentration of montelukast by about 40%.

- Montelukast with statins such as atorvastatin or simvastatin poses a moderate risk of peripheral neuropathy, which is characterized by tingling, burning, pain, or numbness in the hands and feet.
- It is not known whether montelukast interacts with herbal remedies designed to treat allergy symptoms.

Tell Your Doctor
- If you have any allergies and all OTC and prescription medications you are taking, as well as supplements.
- If you have phenylketonuria (PKU), because the chewable tablets contain aspartame that forms phenylalanine.
- If you have liver disease.

Of Special Interest to Women
- Montelukast crosses the placenta after oral use in animals, but it is not known whether the same occurs in pregnant women. Your doctor may prescribe montelukast if he or she feels the benefits outweigh the potential but unknown risks to the fetus.
- Studies in animals show that montelukast is excreted in milk, but it is not known whether the same occurs in humans.

Symptoms of Overdose
Headache, restlessness or agitation, sleepiness, stomach pain, thirst, and vomiting.

Neostigmine Bromide

Brand Name
Prostigmin
Available as Generic?
No
Principal Use
Myasthenia gravis
About the Drug
Neostigmine bromide is prescribed to improve muscle strength in people who have myasthenia gravis. The drug prevents the breakdown of acetylcholine, a natural substance that is necessary for normal muscle function.
How to Use This Drug
Neostigmine is available as tablets for oral use and via injection (the parenteral form, neostigmine methylsulfate) if swallowing and/or breath-

ing is a problem. The daily oral dose varies from 15 mg to 375 mg, with an average of 10 tablets (150 mg) over a 24-hour period. The interval between each dose is very important, and your doctor will determine the best schedule for you and adjust it as needed.

It is very important that you use neostigmine exactly as prescribed by your health-care provider. He or she may ask you to keep a daily record of when you take the drug and how long it is effective. This information can help your doctor make adjustments to your dose as needed.

Side Effects

- Most common side effects: abdominal cramps, diarrhea, decreased pupil size, increased sweating, increased saliva, increased urination, nausea, and vomiting.
- Less common but serious side effects: abnormal heartbeat, dizziness, headache, new or increased muscle cramps, weakness or twitching, new or increased difficulty swallowing, seizures, and shortness of breath. Contact your doctor immediately if these occur.

Possible Drug, Supplement, and/or Food Interactions

- Certain antibiotics, especially kanamycin, neomycin, and streptomycin, should be used only when definitely indicated and you are monitored closely.
- Local and general anesthetics, antiarrhythmic agents (e.g., metoprolol, propranolol, quinidine), and other drugs that interfere with neuromuscular transmission should be used with caution and avoided if possible.
- The following drugs may cause adverse effects if taken with neostigmine, so be sure you tell your doctor if you are using any of them: atropine, belladonna, clidinium, dicyclomine, glycopyrrolate, hyoscyamine, mepenzolate, methantheline, methscopolamine, propantheline, scopolamine.

Tell Your Doctor

- If you have any allergies, especially a history of reaction to bromides.
- All prescription and OTC medications you are using, as well as supplements.
- If you have asthma, blood vessel or circulation problems, epilepsy or other seizure disorders, heart rhythm disorder, overactive thyroid (hyperthyroidism), peritonitis or obstruction of the intestinal or urinary tract, peptic ulcer, or vagotonia.
- If you plan to have surgery, including dental surgery, tell your surgeon or dentist that you are taking neostigmine.

Of Special Interest to Women
- Neostigmine is a pregnancy Category C drug, which means there are no adequate or well-controlled studies in animals or pregnant women. This drug should be used only if your health-care provider believes it is clearly needed.
- It is not known whether neostigmine is excreted in breast milk. Consult your health-care provider about the benefits and risks of breast-feeding while taking this medication.
- Neostigmine may cause uterine irritability and induce premature labor when pregnant women take it near term.

Symptoms of Overdose

A cholinergic crisis, which is characterized by increasing muscle weakness, which can eventually affect the muscles necessary for breathing and result in death. A myasthenic crisis is also characterized by extreme muscle weakness, so it can be difficult to distinguish between a cholinergic crisis and an increase in the severity of myasthenia gravis. It is critical that you see your health-care provider immediately if you experience increasing muscle weakness.

Omega-3 Fatty Acids

See Fish Oil Supplements

Oxycodone

Brand Names

ETH-Oxydose, M-oxy, Oxyfast, OxyIR, OxyContin, Roxicodone

Available as Generic?

Yes

Principal Use

Moderate to severe pain

About the Drug

Oxycodone is a potent narcotic pain reliever and cough suppressant that is similar to codeine, hydrocodone, and morphine. Although experts have not identified its exact mechanism of action, they believe it works by stimulating opioid receptors in the brain. This results in an increase in your tolerance to pain but does not eliminate the sensation of pain.

Oxycodone has a high potential to cause physical and psychological dependence, and its drug class (narcotic pain relievers) is among the most abused in the United States. The risk of addiction is higher if you are or have previously abused other drugs or alcohol.

How to Use This Drug

Oxycodone is available as both immediate- and controlled-release tablets and as an oral concentrate solution. The initial dose of the immediate-release tablets is 5–30 mg every 4 hours. If it is your first time taking an opioid, your initial dose will likely be 5–15 mg every 4–6 hours.

For the controlled-release tablets, the typical starting dose is 10 mg every 12 hours. Do not crush, chew, or break the tablets; swallow them whole. If the tablets are broken in any way, it causes a rapid release of the drug, which can be dangerous.

Higher-dose tablets (60, 80, and 160 mg) or single doses that exceed 40 mg should be used only if you have been taking opioids and are tolerant to opioid treatment. If you are not used to taking opioids, large doses may cause depressed breathing.

The oral concentrate solution is available in two formulations. The usual dose of the 5 mg/mL solution is 10–30 mg every 4 hours; the usual dose for the 20 mg/mL solution is 5 mg every 6 hours. Be sure to use the special measuring device provided with the prescription; do not use a household spoon because it will give you an incorrect amount of the medication.

If you are taking oxycodone as needed, remember to take it at the first signs of pain. If you wait until your pain worsens, the drug will be less effective.

Side Effects

- Most frequent side effects: constipation, dizziness, dry mouth, headache, light-headedness, nausea, rash, sedation, and sweating.
- Oxycodone can depress your breathing, so it should be used with caution by elderly or fragile individuals and by anyone who has serious lung disease.
- Oxycodone is habit-forming, and mental and physical dependence can occur even with short-term use.
- Symptoms of withdrawal may occur if you suddenly stop taking oxycodone after prolonged use. Consult your doctor and establish a gradual reduction in dose to avoid withdrawal symptoms, which can include diarrhea, irritability, runny nose, stomach cramps, sweating, and trouble sleeping.

Possible Drug, Supplement, and/or Food Interactions

- Oxycodone may increase the risk of serious side effects (e.g., shallow breathing, severe drowsiness or dizziness) if taken with other medications that can also affect breathing or cause drowsiness. These include alcohol, antiseizure drugs, antianxiety drugs (e.g., alprazolam, diazepam), muscle relaxants, other narcotic pain relievers, and psychiatric medicines (e.g., amitriptyline, risperidone). OTC medications may also contain ingredients that cause drowsiness, especially allergy and cold and cough products.
- Oxycodone with antidiarrheal drugs such as diphenoxylate and loperamide can result in severe constipation.
- Drugs that block and stimulate opioid receptors (e.g., buprenorphine, butorphanol, nalbuphine, pentazocine) may reduce the effectiveness of oxycodone and result in withdrawal symptoms.
- Consuming a fatty meal can increase the amount of oxycodone your body absorbs by 27%.
- Oxycodone may interfere with the results of certain lab tests and provide false test results.

Tell Your Doctor

- If you have any allergies, especially to other narcotic pain relievers.
- If you have a history of bowel or intestinal disorders (e.g., colitis, infectious diarrhea), kidney disease, liver disease, lung disease (e.g., asthma, chronic obstructive pulmonary disease), breathing problems (e.g., sleep apnea), certain heart problems (e.g., low blood pressure, irregular heartbeat), personal or family history of alcohol or drug abuse, brain disorders, underactive thyroid, difficulty urinating, pancreatitis, gallbladder disease, adrenal gland disorders, or mental/mood disorders.
- If you plan to have surgery, including dental surgery, tell your doctor or dentist that you are using oxycodone.
- If you have diabetes, alcohol dependence, or liver disease, because the liquid forms of oxycodone may contain sugar and/or alcohol.

Of Special Interest to Women

- Do not use oxycodone during pregnancy unless your doctor has indicated that it is clearly needed. Prolonged or high-dose use of oxycodone near delivery may harm the fetus. Infants born to women who have used oxycodone for an extended period may experience withdrawal symptoms such as irritability, vomiting, diarrhea, and abnormal crying.

- Oxycodone is excreted into breast milk and may cause symptoms in nursing infants. Consult your health-care provider before breast-feeding.

Symptoms of Overdose

Breathing problems, extreme sleepiness, and small pupils.

Paroxetine

Brand Names

Paxil, Paxil CR, Pexeva

Available as Generic?

Yes

Principal Uses

Depression, obsessive-compulsive disorders, panic disorders, post-traumatic stress disorder, premenstrual dysphoric disorder, social anxiety disorder

About the Drug

Paroxetine is a selective serotonin reuptake inhibitor, a class that also contains citalopram (Celexa), fluoxetine (Prozac), and sertraline (Zoloft). Many experts believe depression is caused by an imbalance among neurotransmitters (chemicals that facilitate communication among nerve cells in the brain). SSRIs work by helping to restore the balance of neurotransmitters. Specifically, paroxetine prevents the reuptake of the neurotransmitter serotonin by nerve cells after it has been released by nerves in the brain, which in turn increases the amount of free serotonin to stimulate nerve cells and thus helps prevent depressive symptoms.

How to Use This Drug

Paroxetine is available as immediate-release tablets, controlled-release tablets, and suspension. The recommended dose is 20–60 mg daily of the immediate-release tablets or 12.5–75 mg of the controlled-release tablets. If you take paroxetine with food, you may reduce your risk of nausea, a common side effect.

Like other antidepressants, you will not experience the full effect of the drug for a few weeks. Dosing for obsessive-compulsive disorders and panic disorders tends to be higher than for depression. If you are taking paroxetine for premenstrual problems, your health-care provider may prescribe it every day or just for the 2 weeks before your period until the first full day of your period.

If you are older than 65, in poor health, or have certain kidney or liver diseases, your doctor may lower your dose to avoid toxic levels of the drug in your system.

Side Effects

- Common side effects: anxiety, constipation, diarrhea, drowsiness, dry mouth, headache, insomnia, loss of appetite, nausea, sweating, and weakness.
- Less common side effects: high blood pressure, seizures, and sexual dysfunction.
- Severe and unlikely side effects that should be reported immediately to your doctor: black/tarry stools, blurry vision, change in urine output, easy bruising or bleeding, fainting, fast or irregular heartbeat, muscle weakness or spasms, numbness or tingling, restlessness, severe or unusual mental/mood changes (e.g., thoughts of suicide, agitation), tremors, or vomit that looks like coffee grounds.
- Stopping paroxetine suddenly may cause withdrawal symptoms such as anxiety, insomnia, mood swings, nausea, nervousness, and "shock-like" feelings. Talk to your doctor about how to taper off.
- An increased risk of suicidal thinking and behaviors has been noted in young individuals (up to about age 25) during the early stages of taking paroxetine.
- Paroxetine rarely causes serotonin syndrome, a very serious condition characterized by fast heartbeat, hallucinations, loss of coordination, severe diarrhea, severe nausea/vomiting, twitchy muscles, and unexplained fever.

Possible Drug, Supplement, and/or Food Interactions

- Paroxetine with any of the following medications increases your risk of the rare but very serious condition serotonin syndrome: triptans (e.g., eletriptan, sumatriptan), certain antidepressants including other SSRIs (e.g., citalopram, fluoxetine), and SNRIs (e.g., duloxetin, venlafaxine), lithium, tramadol, tryptophan, and sibutramine.
- Paroxetine should not be taken with MAOI antidepressants, including isocarboxazid, phenelzine, tranylcypromine, selegiline, and procarbazine. A 14-day period without treatment should occur when switching between paroxetine and MAOIs.
- Paroxetine should not be taken with other drugs that increase serotonin in the brain, including meperdine, tramadol, and tryptophan, and the herb Saint-John's-wort.
- Paroxetine with aspirin and NSAIDs or other drugs that affect

bleeding may increase the occurrence of upper gastrointestinal bleeding.

- Paroxetine with warfarin and other blood thinners (e.g., aspirin, clopidogrel) may lead to excessive bleeding.
- Drugs that can cause drowsiness should be used with caution and your doctor's approval. These include certain antihistamines (e.g., diphenhydramine), antiseizure drugs (e.g., carbamazepine), medications for sleep or anxiety (e.g., alprazolam, diazepam), muscle relaxants, narcotic pain relievers, psychiatric medications (e.g., nortriptyline, quetiapine).
- Phenytoin and phenobarbital may decrease the amount of paroxetine in the body and reduce its effectiveness.
- Cimetidine is a common OTC heartburn drug that can cause undesirable interactions with paroxetine. Consult your doctor or pharmacist about other treatments for heartburn.
- Avoid use of alcohol while taking paroxetine.

Tell Your Doctor
- If you have any allergies, and all prescription and OTC medications you are taking, as well as supplements.
- If you have a personal or family history of bipolar/manic-depressive disorder or of suicide attempts.
- If you have liver problems, kidney disease, low sodium in the blood, glaucoma (narrow-angle type), seizures, dehydration, or stomach or intestinal ulcers.

Of Special Interest to Women
- Use of paroxetine during pregnancy has been linked to congenital heart defects. Discuss the use of alternative antidepressant treatment during pregnancy with your health-care provider.
- Paroxetine passes into breast milk. Consult your health-care provider about alternative treatments and the benefits and risks of breast-feeding while taking paroxetine.
- Babies born to a mother who used paroxetine during the last trimester may develop withdrawal symptoms such as feeding difficulties, breathing problems, seizures, muscle stiffness, or constant crying. Contact your health-care provider promptly if your infant has these symptoms.

Symptoms of Overdose
Fainting, irregular heartbeat, seizures, and severe dizziness.

Prednisone

Brand Names

Cortan, Deltasone, Liquid Pred, Meticorten, Orasone, Prednicen-M, Sterapred

Available as Generic?

Yes

Principal Uses

Rheumatoid arthritis, gouty arthritis, polymyositis, psoriatic arthritis, severe psoriasis, lupus, bronchial asthma, contact dermatitis

About the Drug

Prednisone is a corticosteroid hormone (glucocorticoid) that reduces the immune system's response to a variety of diseases such as arthritis, blood disorders, breathing problems, certain cancers, eye problems, immune system diseases, and skin disorders. Although prednisone can be helpful in treating symptoms of a variety of diseases and disorders, it also suppresses the immune system and makes you more susceptible to infection or can worsen an infection you already have or recently had.

How to Use This Drug

Prednisone is available in tablets and liquid. Take it with a full glass of water and with food to help prevent stomach upset. If your doctor has prescribed once-a-day dosing, you will likely take that dose before 9 A.M. each day. Sometimes dosing is scheduled for every other day or on another schedule, per your doctor's instructions. If you use the liquid form, use the measuring device supplied with the medication; do not use a household spoon.

It may take several days or longer, depending on your condition, before you notice the benefits of prednisone. Do not suddenly stop taking prednisone, as you may experience a worsening of symptoms. Your doctor can tell you how to gradually reduce your dose to avoid adverse events.

Side Effects

- Common side effects: dizziness, headache, stomach upset, and trouble sleeping.
- Unlikely but serious side effects that should be reported to your healthcare provider: abdominal pain, black stools, bone pain, breathing difficulties, coffee-ground vomit, easy bruising or bleeding, heartburn,

increased thirst and urination, irregular or pounding heartbeat, menstrual period changes, mental/mood changes, muscle pain or weakness, persistent weight gain, puffy face, seizures, signs of infection (e.g., fever, persistent sore throat), swelling of the ankles or feet, and vision changes.

Possible Drug, Supplement, and/or Food Interactions

- Prednisone with aldesleukin or natalizumab may cause very serious interactions.
- The following drugs may cause troublesome interactions with prednisone: aspirin and aspirinlike drugs (e.g., salicylates), birth control pills, blood thinners (e.g., warfarin), mifepristone, NSAIDs that decrease potassium levels (e.g., ampotericin B), drugs that affect certain liver enzymes (CYP3A4 substrates such as azole antifungals, macrolide antibiotics).
- Prednisone may interact with estrogens, resulting in an increase in the levels of the active form of prednisone, prednisolone, in the body and thus lead to more frequent side effects.
- Phenytoin can reduce the effectiveness of prednisone.
- Avoid immunizations, skin tests, and vaccinations while taking prednisone unless you are specifically directed by your health-care provider.
- Prednisone may interfere with certain lab tests (including skin tests) and cause false test results.
- Prednisone may increase your blood sugar levels.

Tell Your Doctor

- About any allergies and all prescription and OTC medications you are taking, as well as supplements (especially Saint-John's-wort).
- If you have any untreated active fungal infections, other infections, bleeding problems, history of blood clots, diabetes, eye conditions (e.g., cataracts, glaucoma), heart problems, high blood pressure, kidney disease, history of malaria, mental/mood conditions, myasthenia gravis, osteoporosis, severe liver disease, stomach or intestinal problems, or an underactive thyroid.
- If you have taken prednisone in the past.
- If you are planning to undergo surgery.
- If you are exposed to chicken pox or measles infection while taking prednisone, contact your doctor immediately.
- If you experience unusual stress, such as illness, surgery, or a medical emergency, as your prednisone dose may need to be adjusted.

Of Special Interest to Women

- Prednisone should be used during pregnancy only if your doctor believes it is necessary, as there have been rare reports of harm to the fetus.
- Infants born to women who have taken prednisone during pregnancy have had low levels of corticosteroid hormone. Symptoms of affected infants may include severe diarrhea, persistent nausea or vomiting, and weakness.
- Prednisone passes into breast milk. Although there are no reports of harm to nursing infants, consult with your health-care provider before you breast-feed.
- Prednisone may increase your risk of developing osteoporosis. Talk to your doctor about how to prevent this bone loss disease.

Symptoms of Overdose

A single large dose of prednisone typically does not cause life-threatening symptoms. Long-term use of high doses of prednisone, however, may cause changes in the location and shape of body fat (especially in the face, back, neck, and waist), easy bruising, increased acne or facial hair, loss of interest in sex, and menstrual problems.

Pregabalin

Brand Name

Lyrica

Available as Generic?

No

Principal Uses

Pain caused by neurologic diseases such as postherpetic neuralgia (pain after shingles) and diabetic neuropathy; also for seizures and fibromyalgia

About the Drug

Pregabalin is an anticonvulsant medication that is chemically related to gabapentin (Neurontin). Its mechanism of action is uncertain; however, it binds to calcium channels on nerves and may change the release of chemicals (neurotransmitters) that nerves use to communicate with each other. By reducing the signals that pass between nerves, pregabalin may help reduce pain and seizures.

How to Use This Drug

Pregabalin is available as capsules and as an oral solution. You may take pregabalin with or without food. Dosing depends on your condition and what your health-care provider prescribes. Generally, the initial dose for neuropathic pain is 50 mg 3 times daily, and this dose may be increased to a maximum of 100 mg 3 times daily after 1 week.

For postherpetic neuralgia, the typical initial dose is 75 mg twice daily or 50 mg 3 times daily. Dosing may be increased to 100 mg 3 times daily after 1 week. If this dose does not provide sufficient pain relief after 2–4 weeks of treatment, your health-care provider may increase your dose to 300 mg twice daily or 200 mg 3 times daily.

For fibromyalgia, the dose is typically 300–450 mg daily in 2 or 3 divided doses. For seizures, the initial dose is usually 150 mg daily and then increased gradually based on your response to a maximum of 600 mg daily.

Side Effects

- Most common side effects: blurry vision, difficulty concentrating, dizziness, dry mouth, sleepiness, swelling of hands and feet, and weight gain.
- Other side effects: reduced blood platelet count and increased blood creatinine kinase levels.
- Anticonvulsant medications like pregabalin have been associated with an increased risk of suicidal thoughts and behaviors.

Possible Drug, Supplement, and/or Food Interactions

- Drinking alcohol may increase the sedative effects of pregabalin.
- Pregabalin with pioglitazone or rosiglitazone may increase fluid retention and weight gain.
- Pregabalin with other drugs that have a sedative effect can increase sleepiness.
- Your chance of experiencing swelling and hives increases if you take ACE inhibitors with pregabalin.
- Narcotic pain medications such as oxycodone, tranquilizers, or anti-anxiety drugs (e.g., lorazepam) with pregabalin may increase dizziness and sleepiness.

Tell Your Doctor

- If you have or have ever had depression, mood problems, or suicidal thoughts or behaviors.
- If you have kidney problems; heart problems; bleeding disorders or a low blood platelet count; or if you have ever had swelling of your face, mouth, tongue, lips, gums, neck, or throat.
- If you have ever abused prescription medications, alcohol, or street drugs.

Of Special Interest to Women
- No adequate studies of the impact of pregabalin in pregnant women have been done. Discuss the benefits and risks of taking this drug with your physician.
- It is not known whether pregabalin is excreted in breast milk. Discuss the benefits and risks of using pregabalin if you are breast-feeding.
- If you become pregnant while taking pregabalin, talk to your doctor about the North American Antiepileptic Drug Pregnancy Registry. The registry collects information about the safety of antiepileptic drugs during pregnancy. 1-888-233-2334.

Symptoms of Overdose
Not known. Doses as high as 8000 mg have not caused problems except for the usual side effects.

Raloxifene

Brand Name
Evista

Available as Generic?
No

Principal Uses
Osteoporosis (prevention and treatment); to decrease the risk of developing invasive breast cancer in women at high risk of developing this cancer or who have osteoporosis

About the Drug
Raloxifene is in the drug class selective estrogen receptor modulators (SERMs). For the prevention and treatment of osteoporosis, raloxifene works by mimicking the effects of the hormone estrogen to increase the thickness (density) of bone. For women who are at high risk of developing invasive breast cancer, raloxifene blocks the impact of estrogen on breast tissue, which may stop the development of hormone-dependent tumors. Raloxifene cannot be used to reduce the risk of developing noninvasive breast cancer, to treat invasive breast cancer, or to prevent invasive breast cancer from recurring.

How to Use This Drug
Raloxifene is available as tablets that are usually taken once daily with or without food. The typical dose is 60 mg. To get the most benefit from raloxifene, be sure to include foods that are rich in calcium and vitamin D in your diet daily to help support bone strength.

Side Effects

- Common side effects: hot flashes, leg cramps, and sweating. If these worsen or persist, contact your physician.
- Less common but serious side effects: changes in or problems with vision; confusion; coughing up blood; feeling of warmth in the lower leg; leg pain; severe headache; shortness of breath; sudden chest pain; or swelling of the hands, feet, ankles, or lower legs. Contact your physician immediately if any of these occur.

Possible Drug, Supplement, and/or Food Interactions

- If you are taking any of the following medications, your health-care provider may need to change your doses or monitor you for side effects: anticoagulants (e.g., warfarin), cholestyramine, colestipol, diazepam, diazoxide, estrogens (e.g., ERT, HRT), estrogen blockers (e.g., letrozole), and lidocaine.
- Raloxifene may affect the results of certain lab tests. Tell your health-care provider and lab personnel that you are taking this drug.

Tell Your Doctor

- If you have any allergies and all prescription and OTC medications you take, as well as supplements.
- If you have a history of blood clots in your legs, lungs, or eyes, raloxifene may increase your risk of developing a blood clot in your lungs or legs. Your doctor will not prescribe raloxifene for you.
- If you have any type of cancer, breast lumps, kidney disease, liver disease, high blood pressure, heart or blood vessel disease, stroke, high cholesterol, or a history of high triglycerides due to estrogen treatment.
- If you develop vaginal bleeding or spotting while taking raloxifene, or if you notice breast tenderness, enlargement, or lumps.
- If you are planning to undergo any type of surgery. Your doctor will instruct you to stop using raloxifene at least 3 days before the procedure. Do not begin taking it again until you consult with your doctor.

Of Special Interest to Women

- Raloxifene should not be used unless you have gone through menopause and cannot get pregnant. However, if you become pregnant, contact your health-care provider immediately, as raloxifene may harm the fetus.
- Although it is not known whether raloxifene passes into breast milk, it is recommended that you not breast-feed.

- During long periods of inactivity, such as prolonged travel, make sure you move around periodically to keep your blood flowing and to prevent blood clots.
- Your doctor may recommend that you periodically undergo bone density tests and/or blood mineral level testing to monitor your progress. He or she may also recommend that you eat and drink foods and beverages rich in calcium and vitamin D and/or recommend a supplement.
- In one trial, there was an increased risk of death due to stroke in postmenopausal women who had coronary heart disease or who were at increased risk for a major coronary event, such as heart attack.

Symptoms of Overdose
Leg cramps and dizziness.

Risedronate

Brand Name
Actonel
Available as Generic?
No
Principal Uses
Prevention and treatment of osteoporosis, treatment of Paget's disease
About the Drug
Risedronate is a bisphosphonate, a drug class that also includes alendronate (Fosamax), etidronate (Didronel, not approved by the FDA for osteoporosis), ibandronate (Boniva), and zoledronic (Reclast). This drug works by slowing down the rate at which bone is dissolved. Unlike the other bisphosphonates, risedronate has a chemically unique component that is believed to reduce gastrointestinal side effects, and it also is more effective at blocking the loss of bone than alendronate and etidronate.
How to Use This Drug
Risedronate is available in tablets and must be taken after getting up in the morning and before eating, drinking, or taking other medications. Take risedronate with a full glass of plain water and not with any other beverage. Swallow the tablet whole; do not chew or suck on it. You must remain fully upright (sitting, walking, standing) for at least 30 minutes after you take the medication. During that 30-minute period, do not eat or drink anything (plain water is okay), and do not take any other medi-

cations or supplements. After 30 minutes, you may eat, drink, or take any other medications or supplements unless directed otherwise by your health-care provider. Do not lie down until after you have had your first food of the day.

The usual dose of risedronate for osteoporosis is 5 mg once daily, one 35 mg tablet once weekly, one 75 mg tablet taken on 2 consecutive days in a month, or one 150 mg tablet taken once a month. For Paget's disease, your doctor may prescribe 30 mg daily for 2 months.

Ask your health-care provider what you should do if you forget to take a dose of your medication. If you do not take risedronate exactly as your doctor prescribed, do not take it any other time during the day.

Side Effects

- Common side effects: abdominal pain (11% of patients), diarrhea (20%), headache (20%), joint pain (33%), nausea (10%), and rash (11%).
- Less likely but serious side effects: bone, joint, or muscle pain; jaw pain; vision problems. Contact your health-care provider if these side effects occur.
- Serious side effects that should be reported immediately to your health-care provider: black/tarry stools, chest pain, difficult or painful swallowing, severe stomach pain, or vomit that looks like coffee grounds.
- Risedronate infrequently causes irritation and ulcers of the esophagus or stomach.
- Infrequently, a serious jawbone problem (osteonecrosis) has occurred in people who have taken medications similar to risedronate.

Possible Drug, Supplement, and/or Food Interactions

- Certain foods and supplements may interfere with absorption of risedronate, including calcium and iron supplements; vitamins with minerals; antacids that contain calcium, magnesium, or aluminum; dairy products; and calcium-enriched juice. Do not take any of these products for at least 30 minutes after you take risedronate.
- Medications such as quinapril, sucralfate, and bismuth subsalicylate may interfere with absorption of risedronate. Do not take these products for at least 30 minutes after taking risedronate.
- Aspirin or NSAIDs such as ibuprofen with risedronate may increase the risk of stomach irritation or ulcers. The same is true for other medications, such as cold or flu products, that include these ingredients. However, if your doctor has prescribed low-dose aspirin for a specific medical reason such as stroke or heart attack prevention,

continue to take the aspirin, but consult with your doctor as a pre-caution.

- Risedronate may affect the results of some lab tests, so tell your health-care provider and lab personnel that you are using this drug.

Tell Your Doctor
- If you have any allergies, and all prescription and OTC medications you are taking, as well as supplements.
- If you have any mouth or dental problems that need attention, take care of them before starting risedronate. Give your dentist your complete medical history, including medication use and whether you have ever had cancer radiation treatments.
- If you have the following conditions: low blood calcium levels, an inability to remain upright for at least 30 minutes, kidney disease, esophagus problems, difficult or painful swallowing, cancer, anemia, blood-clotting disorders, or gastrointestinal disorders.

Of Special Interest to Women
- Risedronate can stay in the body for many years, and its effects on the fetus are not known. If you get pregnant, discuss the benefits and risks of taking risedronate with your health-care provider.
- It is not known whether risedronate passes into breast milk. Consult your health-care provider before breast-feeding.

Symptoms of Overdose
Muscle spasms, numbness, seizures, and tingling sensations. You can drink milk after an overdose to help reduce absorption of the drug while you are waiting for medical assistance.

Simvastatin

Brand Name
Zocor
Available as Generic?
Yes
Principal Uses
High cholesterol; to reduce risk of death in patients with cardiovascular disease, diabetes
About the Drug
Simvastatin is a cholesterol-lowering drug that belongs to a drug class called statins. Other drugs in this class include atorvastatin (Lipitor), fluvastatin (Lescol), lovastatin (Mevacor), rosuvastatin (Crestor). Sim-

vastatin reduces cholesterol and fats (triglycerides) in the blood by inhibiting the action of an enzyme in the liver (HMG-CoA reductase) needed to make cholesterol. It can also raise high-density lipoprotein ("good" HDL) levels, which may slow coronary artery disease. In 2009, simvastatin was the second most popular drug in the United States, where it was prescribed 83 million times, according to an IMS Health report.

How to Use This Drug

Simvastatin is available in regular and disintegrating tablets. The typical starting dose is 20–40 mg once daily, while the dose range is 5–80 mg per day, usually taken in the evening. If you have familial hypercholesterolemia, your doctor may instruct you to take simvastatin more frequently. You can take simvastatin with or without food.

Take simvastatin at the same time each day. It may take up to 1 month before you get the most benefit from this drug. For best results, simvastatin should be used along with regular exercise, a low-fat, low-cholesterol diet, and a weight-loss program if you are overweight.

Side Effects

- Most common side effects: abdominal pain, abnormal liver tests, diarrhea, headache, muscle pain, nausea, and vomiting.
- Serious, less likely side effects: liver damage and a condition called rhabdomyolysis that is characterized by muscle breakdown or inflammation. Rhabdomyolysis causes the release of the protein myoglobin into the blood, and this protein can lead to kidney failure or death. When used alone, statins cause rhabdomyolysis in less than 1% of patients.

Possible Drug, Supplement, and/or Food Interactions

- Grapefruit juice and grapefruit can increase the amount of simvastatin in your bloodstream.
- Take simvastatin at least 1 hour before or at least 2 hours after other drugs that lower cholesterol (bile acid–binding resins), such as cholestyramine or colestipol.
- All of the following drugs can reduce elimination of simvastatin, increase the risk of muscle toxicity, and even cause fatal interactions: some azole antifungals (e.g., itraconazole, ketoconazole), delavirdine, HIV protease inhibitors (e.g., amprenavir, ritonavir), some macrolide antibiotics (e.g., clarithromycin, erythromycin), nefazodone, telithromycin.
- Simvastatin with the following medications and supplements may increase the risk of muscle toxicity (e.g., cramps, pain), although your health-care provider can make dose adjustments and monitor you

carefully: warfarin, danazol, daptomycin, digoxin, drugs that affect certain liver enzymes (e.g., amiodarone, cyclosporine, diltiazem, verapamil), and the herb Saint-John's-wort.

- Daily use of alcohol increases your risk of serious side effects.

Tell Your Doctor

- If you have any allergies, especially to other statins, and all OTC and prescription medications you are taking, as well as supplements.
- If you have active liver disease, as you should not be using this medication.
- If you have a history of alcohol use, kidney disease, or liver disease.
- If you plan to have surgery, including dental surgery, tell your doctor or dentist you are taking simvastatin.

Of Special Interest to Women

- Do not use simvastatin during pregnancy. The drug reduces cholesterol, a substance necessary for development of the fetus.
- Simvastatin while breast-feeding may harm your infant, so do not use this drug.

Symptoms of Overdose

None expected to cause life-threatening symptoms.

Solifenacin

Brand Name

VESicare

Available as Generic?

No

Principal Use

Overactive bladder

About the Drug

Solifenacin belongs to the drug class anticholinergics, and is also referred to as an antispasmodic. The drug works by relaxing the muscles in the bladder (antispasm), which improves your ability to control urination, such as leakage, an urgent need to urinate, and frequent trips to the bathroom.

How to Use This Drug

Solifenacin is available in tablets and can be taken with or without food. It is usually dosed once daily, unless your doctor gives you other instructions. He or she will likely start you on a low dose and then increase it if necessary over time.

Take solifenacin with a full glass of liquid and at the same time each day. Do not split, crush, or chew the tablets; take them whole.

Side Effects

- Common side effects: blurry vision, dry eyes, constipation, stomach pain or upset, and unusual tiredness or weakness.
- Infrequent but serious side effects: constipation that lasts for 3 or more days, severe abdominal pain, urination difficulties, and signs of kidney infection (e.g., burning or painful urination, lower back pain, fever).
- Serious allergic reactions are rare, but seek immediate medical help if you experience rash, itching/swelling (especially of the face, tongue, and/or throat), severe dizziness, and breathing difficulties.
- Solifenacin may make it more difficult for your body to cool down when it gets very hot. Symptoms of heat stroke include confusion, dizziness, fast pulse, fever, headache, and upset stomach. Seek immediate medical assistance.

Possible Drug, Supplement, and/or Food Interactions

- Solifenacin with pramlintide can result in very serious interactions.
- Solifenacin may interact with the following medications and supplements: amiodarone, antifungals such as fluconazole and itraconazole, carbamazepine, cimetidine, cisapride, clarithromycin, cyclosporine, danazol, delavirdine, dexamethasone, diltiazem, disopyramide, dofetilide, erythromycin, ethosuximide, fluoxetine, fluvoxamine, HIV protease inhibitors such as indinavir and ritonavir, isoniazid, metronidazole, moxifloxacin, nefazodone, other antispasmodics such as dicyclomine, phenobarbital, potassium tablets or capsules, quinidine, rifampin, sotalol, thioridazine, verapamil, zafirlukast, and the herb Saint-John's-wort. Your doctor may need to alter your doses or monitor you closely.
- Limit alcohol use when taking solifenacin.
- Do not drink grapefruit juice or eat grapefruit while taking solifenacin.

Tell Your Doctor

- If you have any allergies to medications, supplements (especially Saint-John's-wort), preservatives, or additives, including corn.
- About all OTC and prescription medications you are taking.
- If you or anyone in your family has or ever had prolonged QT interval, a heart problem in which an electrical malfunction can cause fainting.
- If you have difficulty emptying your bladder (urinary retention), severe liver disease, uncontrolled narrow-angle glaucoma,

or severe blockage of your stomach or intestines (gastric retention). You should not use solifenacin if you have any of these conditions.

- If you have a history of bladder problems, stomach and/or intestinal disease, controlled narrow-angle glaucoma, severe constipation, kidney disease, or myasthenia gravis.
- If you are pregnant, plan to get pregnant, or are breast-feeding.
- If you are planning surgery, including dental surgery, tell your doctor or dentist that you are taking solifenacin.

Of Special Interest to Women
- If you are elderly, you may be more sensitive to this drug; it is removed by the kidneys, and kidney function declines with age.
- Solifenacin should not be used during pregnancy unless your doctor decides it's necessary.
- It is not known whether solifenacin is excreted into breast milk. Consult your doctor before breast-feeding.

Symptoms of Overdose
A fast or irregular heartbeat and agitation.

Spironolactone

Brand Name
Aldactone

Available as Generic?
Yes

Principal Uses
High blood pressure; fluid retention caused by heart disease, liver disease, or kidney disease; also myasthenia gravis

About the Drug
Spironolactone is a diuretic (water pill) prescribed to treat high blood pressure and fluid retention. It is also used to treat excessive hair growth in women who have polycystic ovary disease. Spironolactone works by removing excess fluid from the body through urination. However, because it is a potassium-sparing diuretic, it does not deplete the body of necessary potassium.

How to Use This Drug
Spironolactone is available as tablets that are usually taken once daily in the morning, or twice daily. It is recommended you take spironolactone

before 6 P.M. (or at least 3–4 hours before you go to bed) to avoid having to get up often during the night to urinate. It takes about 2 weeks for you to notice the benefits of spironolactone.

Side Effects

- Common side effects: diarrhea, dizziness, drowsiness, dry mouth, enlarged breasts, headache, increased hair growth on the body, irregular menstrual periods, restlessness, stomach pain or cramps, thirst, unsteadiness, vaginal bleeding in postmenopause, and vomiting.
- Less common side effects that should be reported to your health-care provider immediately: blurry vision, breathing difficulties, changes in heartbeat, confusion, decreased urination, extreme tiredness, fever, flulike symptoms, hives, inability to move your arms or legs, itching, loss of appetite, muscle weakness or cramps, nausea, pain or burning in the hands or feet, swallowing difficulties, unusual bleeding or bruising, vomiting blood, or yellowing of the eyes or skin.

Possible Drug, Supplement, and/or Food Interactions

- Talk to your doctor about how much potassium you can safely have in your diet while you are taking this medication. Avoid potassium-containing salt substitutes, and you may need to limit potassium-rich foods such as bananas, raisins, and orange juice.
- Spironolactone with other medications that may increase your potassium levels could make your potassium levels too high (symptoms: irregular heartbeat, nausea. These drugs include ACE inhibitors (e.g., captopril, lisinopril), amiloride, candesartan, cyclosporine, losartan, potassium supplements, tacrolimus, and triamterene.

Tell Your Doctor

- If you have any allergies and all OTC and prescription medications you are taking, as well as supplements.
- If you have kidney disease, liver disease, or high blood potassium (hyperkalemia).
- If you plan to have surgery, including dental surgery, tell your doctor or dentist you are taking spironolactone.

Of Special Interest to Women

- If you are pregnant or become pregnant while taking spironolactone, contact your health-care provider immediately. Spironolactone should be used only when clearly needed during pregnancy.
- Do not breast-feed if you are taking spironolactone because this drug breaks down into other substances that pass into breast milk.

Symptoms of Overdose

Cold skin, confusion, diarrhea, dizziness, drowsiness, irregular heartbeat, lack of energy, loss of muscle tone, nausea, rash, tingling in arms and legs, vomiting, and weakness or heaviness in legs.

Sulfasalazine

Brand Name

Azulfidine

Available as Generic?

Yes

Principal Uses

Ulcerative colitis and rheumatoid arthritis; also ankylosing spondylitis, Crohn's disease

About the Drug

Sulfasalazine is a prodrug, which means it is not active in its oral form. After you take sulfasalazine, bacteria in your colon break it down into 5-aminosalicylic acid (5-ASA) and sulfapyridine. The 5-ASA can reduce inflammation by blocking the activity of prostaglandins, which cause inflammation. Thus sulfasalazine works by reducing swelling and irritation in the large intestinal tract. Delayed-release sulfasalazine tablets are prescribed to treat rheumatoid arthritis, as they help to reduce joint pain, swelling, and stiffness. Sulfasalazine is typically used along with other drugs, rest, and physical therapy in individuals who have not responded to other medications.

How to Use This Drug

Sulfasalazine is available in regular tablets and delayed-release tablets. Take the medication after meals with a full glass of water or as directed by your health-care provider. If you take the delayed-release tablets, do not crush, chew, or break them; take them whole. Dosage of sulfasalazine depends on your body weight, the condition you are being treated for, and how you respond to treatment. Typical adult doses are 1000–4000 mg daily, taken in 2–4 divided doses. For rheumatoid arthritis, it may take 1–3 months before you notice any improvement in symptoms.

If you use the delayed-release tablets and they appear whole or only partly dissolved in your stool, contact your doctor immediately so he or she can change your treatment.

Side Effects

- Common side effects: dizziness, headache, loss of appetite, mouth sores, nausea, stomach upset, unusual tiredness, and vomiting. It may also cause your skin and urine to turn orange-yellow, but this is harmless and will go away when you stop taking the medication.
- Occasionally allergic reactions occur that progress from rash to aching joints and muscles, blistering or peeling skin, fever, problems with swallowing, and unusual weakness and tiredness. Seek medical attention.
- Unlikely but serious side effects you should report immediately to your health-care provider: blood in the urine, change in the amount of urine, painful urination, blurry vision, growth in the neck (goiter), hearing changes, mental/mood changes, numbness or tingling of the hands or feet, rapid heartbeat, or weakness.
- Rarely, potentially dangerous side effects have been reported and include a drop in white blood cell count, anemia characterized by disrupted red blood cells, liver failure, pancreatitis, and kidney failure.

Possible Drug, Supplement, and/or Food Interactions

- Sulfasalazine may reduce the effectiveness of combination-type birth control pills, which can result in pregnancy.
- Serious interactions may occur if you take sulfasalazine with methenamine.
- Sulfasalazine may reduce your body's ability to absorb folic acid and cause folic acid deficiency and anemia.
- Sulfasalazine may reduce the effectiveness of digoxin.
- Sulfasalazine can cause increased blood levels of methotrexate and thus more side effects.
- Sulfasalazine may increase the ability of oral antidiabetic drugs to lower blood glucose levels, resulting in hypoglycemia.
- Sulfasalazine with NSAIDs such as ibuprofen may increase the risk of kidney dysfunction.
- Sulfasalazine and 6-mercaptupurine or azathioprine may increase the risk of blood disorders.
- Sulfasalazine may increase the blood-thinning effect of warfarin.
- Avoid prolonged exposure to the sun, tanning booths, and sunlamps, as sulfasalazine makes you more sensitive to the sun.
- Limit or avoid use of alcohol.

Tell Your Doctor

- If you have any allergies (especially to sulfa drugs, aspirin, salicylates, NSAIDs, or mesalamine) and all OTC and prescription medications you are taking, as well as supplements.

- If you have intestinal blockage, urinary blockage, or the blood disorder porphyria. You should not take sulfasalazine.
- If you have a medical history of blood disorders, kidney disease, liver disease, asthma, severe allergies, or the genetic condition G6PD deficiency.

Of Special Interest to Women

- This drug should be used during pregnancy only if your health-care provider decides it is necessary, because similar drugs may cause harm to infants. Discuss the benefits and risks with your doctor.
- If you are pregnant or plan to get pregnant and are taking sulfasalazine, talk to your doctor about taking folic acid supplements. Sulfasalazine may reduce your folic acid levels, which increases the risk of spinal cord defects in your child.
- Sulfasalazine passes into breast milk and could harm a nursing infant. A by-product of sulfasalazine, called sulfapyridine, may displace bilirubin from albumen in an infant's blood and cause jaundice. Consult your doctor before you breast-feed.

Symptoms of Overdose

Extreme drowsiness, persistent vomiting, seizures, and severe abdominal pain.

Sumatriptan

Brand Names

Alsuma, Imitrex

Available as Generic?

Yes

Principal Use

Migraine

About the Drug

Sumatriptan is a selective serotonin receptor agonist. Other drugs in this class include almotriptan (Axert), eletriptan (Relpax), frovatriptan (Frova), naratriptan (Amerge), rizatriptan (Maxalt), and zolmitriptan (Zomig). Collectively these drugs are sometimes referred to as "triptans."

It is generally believed that migraine headaches occur when blood vessels in the brain dilate (expand). Sumatriptan relieves migraines by stimulating serotonin receptors in the brain, which in turn narrow the blood vessels by prompting the muscles that surround the blood vessels to contract. At the same time, sumatriptan reduces the transmission of pain signals by nerves to the brain. Sumatriptan can relieve migraine pain, but it cannot prevent or reduce the number of headaches.

How to Use This Drug

Sumatriptan is available as tablets, an intranasal spray, and via injection, which you can learn to give to yourself. This medication should be taken with or without food at the first sign of a migraine. If you do not experience improvement in your symptoms after your first dose, do not take any additional doses without speaking with your health-care provider. You should not take more than 200 mg within a 24-hour period.

The oral and intranasal forms of sumatriptan can be used as backup for injections. However, consult your health-care provider about how you should take these additional doses. The recommended oral dose is 25–100 mg, and the maximum dose is 200 mg daily. For the intranasal dose, the recommendation is 5–20 mg, and the maximum is 40 mg daily. If using the injection, the recommended dose is 4 mg or 6 mg injected under the skin, with a maximum daily dose of two 6 mg injections separated by 1 hour.

If you have never taken sumatriptan before and you have risk factors for heart disease, your doctor may ask you to take your first dose in the office to monitor you for rare but serious side effects such as chest pain.

Side Effects

- Common side effects: abdominal discomfort, chest or throat pain or tightness, dizziness, flushing, injection site reactions, nasal irritation, sweating, tingling, and weakness.
- Infrequently, sumatriptan can elevate blood pressure in individuals with or without a history of high blood pressure.
- Rarely, sumatriptan has caused abnormal heartbeat, coronary artery spasm, heart attack, seizures, or stroke.
- Seek immediate medical attention if you experience any of these side effects: bloody diarrhea, chest pain, confusion, fainting, hearing changes, irregular or pounding heartbeat, jaw/left arm pain, mental/mood changes, seizures, slurred speech, sudden or severe abdominal pain, vision changes, or weakness on one side of the body.
- Sumatriptan rarely causes a very serious condition called serotonin syndrome, which is characterized by fast heartbeat, hallucinations, high fever, loss of coordination, severe dizziness, severe nausea/vomiting/diarrhea, twitchy muscles. (See "Possible Drug, Supplement, and/or Food Interactions.")

Possible Drug, Supplement, and/or Food Interactions
- Sumatriptan with other triptans, certain antidepressants (e.g., citalopram, fluoxetine, paroxetine), duloxetine, and venlafaxine can cause a rare condition called serotonin syndrome.
- Monoamine oxidase inhibitors (e.g., isocarboxazid [Marplan], phenelzine [Nardil]) may elevate levels of sumatriptan in the blood and increase side effects. Do not take sumatriptan along with MAOIs or if you have used MAOIs within the previous 2 weeks. Fatal drug interactions are possible.
- Avoid taking sumatriptan within 24 hours of treatment with an ergot-containing medication such as dihydroergotamine or other triptans because the combination increases the risk of vasospasms.
- Sumatriptan with isoniazid, phenothiazines, theophylline, and tricyclic antidepressants (e.g., amitriptyline) may increase your risk of seizures.

Tell Your Doctor
- If you have any allergies, including allergies to other triptan drugs (e.g., rizatriptan, zolmitriptan).
- About all OTC and prescription medications you are taking, as well as supplements.
- If you have any of the following conditions, as you should not take sumatriptan: heart disease, stroke or transient ischemic attack, blood circulation disease, uncontrolled high blood pressure, certain types of headache (e.g., basilar migraine), liver disease.
- If you have certain blood circulation disorders (e.g., Raynaud's disease), diabetes, family history of heart disease, high blood pressure (controlled), high cholesterol, or seizures, or if you smoke.

Of Special Interest to Women
- Sumatriptan should not be taken during pregnancy unless your health-care provider decides it is really necessary.
- Sumatriptan passes into breast milk and may have negative effects on a nursing infant. Exposure of your infant to the drug may be reduced by avoiding breast-feeding for 12 hours after taking sumatriptan. Consult your health-care provider.

Symptoms of Overdose
The same for all forms of the drug: blue-colored lips or fingernails, breathing problems, convulsions, lack of coordination, skin redness, tremors, vision problems, watery eyes or mouth, and weakness.

Tamoxifen

Brand Name

Nolvadex

Available as Generic?

No

Principal Uses

Metastatic breast cancer after radiation or surgery, prevention of invasive breast cancer in women at high risk

About the Drug

Tamoxifen is an antiestrogen drug used to block the growth of breast cancer. Although it is not clear exactly how it works, tamoxifen appears to attach itself to and block estrogen receptors on the surface of cells, which then prevents estrogens from triggering the cells into action.

In addition to the uses listed above, tamoxifen is used to treat women following surgery and radiation who have a less common type of breast cancer called ductal carcinoma in situ. These women are at high risk for developing invasive breast cancer in the future, and tamoxifen can help prevent development of this disease in nearly 50% of women during the first 5 years of treatment. Some physicians prescribe tamoxifen to stimulate ovulation.

How to Use This Drug

Tamoxifen is available as tablets and liquid and can be taken with or without food. If your doctor prescribes more than 20 mg daily, you may take it as a divided dose twice daily. If you are using the liquid form, be sure to use the measuring device provided with the prescription; do not use a household spoon.

Some women experience an increase or flare-up of bone or cancer pain or even new tumors when they begin taking tamoxifen. This may indicate you are responding well to the medication, and the symptoms generally disappear quickly. However, report any symptoms to your health-care provider when they occur.

Side Effects

- Common side effects: abnormal menstrual periods, hot flashes, nausea, thinning hair, and weight gain.
- Unlikely but serious side effects that you should report immediately to your doctor: dark urine, easy bruising or bleeding, eye pain, vision

changes, mental/mood changes, persistent nausea/vomiting, swelling of the ankles or feet, unusual tiredness, and yellowing of the eyes or skin.

- Rarely, tamoxifen has caused very serious and even fatal strokes, blood clots in the lungs or legs, and uterine cancer. Symptoms of stroke or blood clots include calf pain or swelling, chest pain, shortness of breath, slurred speech, and weakness on one side of the body. Symptoms of uterine cancer may include abnormal changes in your period, pain or pressure below your navel, and unusual vaginal discharge.

Possible Drug, Supplement, and/or Food Interactions

- Tamoxifen may cause abnormal results on liver, thyroid, and other blood tests.
- Do not use tamoxifen with anastrozole or letrozole because very serious interactions may occur.
- Some drugs can reduce the effectiveness of tamoxifen, including acetaminophen and combinations (e.g., acetaminophen/diphenhydramine), bupropion, celecoxib, cimetidine, duloxetine, fluoxetine, and paroxetine.
- Some drugs with tamoxifen increase the risk of ventricular arrhythmias, including but not limited to amiodarone, gatifloxacin, and moxifloxacin.
- Tamoxifen with blood thinners such as warfarin increases the risk of serious and fatal hemorrhaging.

Tell Your Doctor

- If you have any allergies and all OTC and prescription medications you are taking, as well as supplements.
- If you have a history of blood clots or any condition that requires you to take blood thinners (e.g., warfarin).
- If your breast cancer is limited to the milk ducts or if you need to take medication to help prevent breast cancer. You should not take tamoxifen.
- If you have cataracts, diabetes, high blood pressure, high cholesterol or triglycerides, limited or no ability to walk, or liver disease, or if you smoke.

Of Special Interest to Women

- Tamoxifen is not recommended for use during pregnancy because it may harm the fetus. Consult your health-care provider immediately if you become pregnant while taking tamoxifen.
- If you are of childbearing age, you will likely start taking tamoxifen during your period or after you get a negative pregnancy test.

It is recommended that you use two effective nonhormonal forms of birth control (e.g., condom plus diaphragm with spermicide) while you take tamoxifen and for 2 months after you stop the drug.

- It is not known whether tamoxifen passes into breast milk. However, because of potential risk to the infant, it is recommended that you not breast-feed.
- Tamoxifen can be absorbed through the skin and breathed into the lungs, so women who are pregnant or who may become pregnant should not handle this medication or breathe in dust from the tablets.

Symptoms of Overdose

Fainting, irregular heartbeat, shaking, and unsteady walking.

Tegaserod

Brand Name

Zelnorm

Available as Generic?

No

Principal Use

Irritable bowel syndrome

About the Drug

Note: Zelnorm was withdrawn from the U.S. market in 2007. However, this medication is still used in limited emergency situations.

Tegaserod increases the activity of serotonin, a chemical in the intestinal tract that speeds the movement of stool through the bowels. It was developed to treat severe, chronic irritable bowel syndrome (IBS) in women whose main bowel complaint is constipation, not diarrhea. Tegaserod can also be used to treat chronic constipation in women who are younger than 55.

How to Use This Drug

Tegaserod is available in tablets, and the usual dose is 6 mg twice daily for 4–12 weeks. It can be taken with or without food, and if taken on an empty stomach, drink a full glass of water. Although this medication is usually taken twice daily, follow your doctor's specific instructions. It can take up to 2 weeks of daily dosing before you notice an improvement in symptoms. Tegaserod is effective only while you are taking it and for up to 1–2 weeks after stopping treatment.

Side Effects
- Most common side effects: headache, migraine, dizziness, back pain, joint pain, mild stomach pain, nausea, gas.
- Serious side effects that should be reported immediately to your doctor: blood in your stools, persistent diarrhea, new and/or worsening severe stomach pain or cramps, feeling like you might pass out.
- Seek emergency care if you experience signs and symptoms of an allergic reaction, which include hives; difficulty breathing; and swelling of your face, lips, tongue, or throat.

Possible Drug, Supplement, and/or Food Interactions

No drug-drug, drug-supplement, or drug-food interactions have been noted for tegaserod. However, any drug or supplement that increases intestinal contractions will probably result in more diarrhea if used with tegaserod.

Tell Your Doctor
- If you have any allergies and all OTC and prescription medications you are taking, as well as supplements.
- If diarrhea is the main problem you are experiencing with IBS, you should not take this drug.
- If you have a history of stroke, heart attack, high blood pressure, uncontrolled angina, high cholesterol, high triglycerides, diabetes, depression, or anxiety, or if you smoke, are overweight, are older than 55, or if you have a history of suicidal thoughts or actions, you should not take tegaserod.
- If you have gallbladder problems, any stomach or intestinal disorders, intestinal blockage, kidney disease, or liver disease, because you may need special tests or dosing.
- If you are breast-feeding, because it is not known whether tegaserod passes into breast milk or if it can affect a nursing infant.

Of Special Interest to Women
- In 2007, the FDA announced that Novartis, the maker of Zelnorm, had agreed to discontinue marketing the drug for the short-term treatment of women who had IBS with constipation and for patients younger than 65 who had chronic constipation. This decision was reached after the FDA's evaluation of safety data from 29 clinical trials that included more than 18,000 patients found an excess number of serious cardiovascular adverse events, including heart attack, stroke, and angina, in patients who took tegaserod compared with those who took placebo.

- The FDA has categorized this drug as Category B, which means it is not expected to be harmful to the fetus. However, tell your doctor if you are pregnant or plan to become pregnant during treatment.

Symptoms of Overdose

Diarrhea, stomach pain, nausea, and vomiting.

Teriparatide

Brand Name

Forteo

Available as Generic?

No

Principal Uses

Osteoporosis in women (and men) with severe osteoarthritis who are at high risk of fractures or already have one or more

About the Drug

Teriparatide is a synthetic form of parathyroid hormone, which is produced naturally by the body. The medication works by increasing bone mass and strength, and thus helps reduce the risk of fracture. Teriparatide is typically administered for several years only, and then patients are switched to another osteoporosis drug, such as alendronate, ibandronate, raloxifene, or zoledronate.

How to Use This Drug

Teriparatide is injected under the skin once daily, usually into the thigh or abdomen. Your doctor or nurse can instruct you how to administer the injection. The medication is available in a multidose prefilled delivery device called a pen. Each pen contains 28 daily doses of 20 mcg.

Teriparatide should be refrigerated between 36° and 46°F; do not freeze, and do not use the medication if it has been frozen. Use the medication immediately after you remove it from the refrigerator and then return it to the refrigerator after use. Recap the pen when you are not using it. Mark the day when you begin using the pen and discard it after 28 days, even if there is still medication in the pen.

Each time you prepare for an injection, check the medication to make sure it is not discolored or has visible particles in it. If either condition exists, do not use the liquid. Clean the injection site with rubbing alcohol, and change your injection site each time to reduce injury under your skin. Use the medication at the same time each day.

Side Effects
- Dizziness or fast heartbeat may occur within 4 hours of injecting the medication. These symptoms may last for a few minutes to a few hours, and typically disappear after several doses as your body adjusts to the medication. Therefore, take the medication while sitting down, be careful when you get up, and avoid driving or other activities that may be dangerous to perform when dizzy.
- Other common side effects: pain, swelling, and/or bruising at the injection site; muscle cramps or spasm.
- Unlikely but serious side effects: constipation, fainting, mental/mood changes, and unusual tiredness.
- Serious allergic reactions are rare. Symptoms include rash; itching and/or swelling of the face, tongue, throat; severe dizziness; and difficulty breathing.

Possible Drug, Supplement, and/or Food Interactions
- Tell your doctor if you are taking digoxin, as you may need a dose adjustment. The two medications together may cause high blood levels of calcium (hypercalcemia).
- Teriparatide may make bisphosphonates less effective.

Tell Your Doctor
- If you have any allergies and all OTC and prescription medications you are using, as well as supplements.
- If you have Paget's disease, if you've had radiation treatment involving your bones, or any other reason you may be at an increased risk for bone tumors. Teriparatide has been shown to increase bone tumors in animals.
- If you have high levels of calcium in your blood (hypercalcemia), kidney stones, or any bone disorders (e.g., bone cancer).

Of Special Interest to Women
- Teriparatide should be used during pregnancy only if your doctor has decided it is clearly needed.
- It is unknown whether teriparatide passes into breast milk. Discuss breast-feeding with your doctor.
- You should undergo periodic lab and/or medical tests to monitor your progress or check for side effects.

Symptoms of Overdose
Nausea, severe dizziness, unusual tiredness, and vomiting.

Tramadol

Brand Names
Ultram, Ultram ER

Available as Generic?
Yes

Principal Uses
Moderate to moderately severe pain, including moderately severe chronic pain that requires continuous treatment for an extended period

About the Drug
Tramadol is a synthetic pain reliever that is similar to morphine in action and is considered a narcotic. Although it is not known exactly how it works, experts believe tramadol binds to opioid receptors in the brain that are responsible for transmitting pain sensations throughout the body. Like other narcotics, tramadol is a frequently abused prescription drug.

How to Use This Drug
Tramadol is available as immediate-release and extended-release tablets and can be taken with or without food. The typical dose is 50–100 mg of the immediate-release tablets every 4–6 hours as needed for pain, with a maximum dose of 400 mg per day. Your doctor will likely start you at 25 mg per day and gradually increase your dose until a safe, effective dose is reached.

Do not chew, crush, or break the extended-release tablets; swallow them whole. The recommended dose is 100 mg daily, with a maximum of 300 mg per day.

Tramadol works best to relieve pain if it is taken at the first sign of pain. If you want to stop taking tramadol, ask your doctor to help you gradually reduce your dose to avoid withdrawal symptoms. Tramadol can lead to addictive behavior and prescription drug abuse.

Side Effects
- Common side effects: constipation, dizziness, drowsiness, headache, nausea, and vomiting.
- Less common side effects: diarrhea, dry mouth, itching, rash, sweating, vertigo, and vision problems.
- Unlikely but serious side effects that you should report immediately to your health-care provider: changes in the amount of urine, extreme stiffness in the muscles, fast heartbeat, loss of coordination,

mental/mood changes, severe abdominal pain, severe nausea/vomiting/diarrhea, unexplained fever, vision changes.

- Abruptly stopping tramadol may cause withdrawal symptoms such as anxiety, diarrhea, hallucinations, insomnia, nausea, pain, rigors, and tremors.

Possible Drug, Supplement, and/or Food Interactions

- Tramadol with alcohol, anesthetics, narcotics, tranquilizers, or sedative hypnotics may increase central nervous system and respiratory depression.
- Drugs that can affect how tramadol works or increase the risk of side effects include azole antifungals (e.g., ketoconazole), carbamazepine, erythromycin, quinidine, rifamycins, and Saint-John's-wort.
- Tramadol with lithium, MAOIs, SSRIs (e.g., citalopram, fluoxetine), SNRIs (e.g., duloxetine), tripans, and other drugs that increase serotonin levels may cause seizures or a potentially fatal condition called serotonin syndrome.
- Drugs such as isoniazid, phenothiazines (e.g., promethazine), theophylline, or tricyclic antidepressants (e.g., amitriptyline) may increase the risk of seizure.

Tell Your Doctor

- If you have any allergies, especially allergies to other narcotics.
- About all OTC and prescription medications you are taking, as well as supplements.
- If you have severe breathing problems, because you should not take this drug.
- If you have any of the following medical conditions: certain bowel diseases (e.g., paralytic ileus), brain disorders (e.g., seizures), metabolic disorders, alcohol or drug withdrawal, adrenal gland problems, heart problems, kidney disease, liver disease, lung diseases, pancreatitis, mental/mood conditions, gastrointestinal disorders (e.g., gallbladder disease), or underactive thyroid.

Of Special Interest to Women

- Tramadol should be used during pregnancy only if it is clearly needed. It is not recommended for long-term use or in high doses late in pregnancy because it may harm the fetus. Infants born to women who have used tramadol for an extended period may experience seizures, abnormal or persistent crying, or diarrhea.
- Tramadol passes into breast milk. Although there are no reports of

harm to nursing infants, consult your health-care provider before you breast-feed.

Symptoms of Overdose

Bluish, clammy skin; coma; extreme lethargy; heart attack; slow, shallow, or stopped breathing; and vomiting. An overdose can be lethal.

Trazodone

Brand Name

Desyrel

Available as Generic?

Yes

Principal Uses

Depression; in combination with other drugs for panic attacks, agoraphobia

About the Drug

Trazodone is an antidepressant that affects the neurotransmitter serotonin, although it is chemically unrelated to other antidepressants that have an impact on serotonin, such as SSRIs. It also is not related to tricyclic antidepressants and MAOIs. Trazodone is related to nefazodone (Serzone) in structure and actions. Although it is not certain exactly how trazodone works, it appears to inhibit the uptake of serotonin by nerves in the brain, which results in more serotonin being available to stimulate other nerves and thus reduce symptoms of depression. In addition to the uses listed above, trazodone is sometimes prescribed to treat insomnia and anxiety.

How to Use This Drug

Trazodone is available in tablets and should be taken after a meal or with a light snack to reduce the risk of dizziness. Taking trazodone with food also increases the amount of the drug your body is able to absorb. Typical doses for depression are 150–600 mg daily, taken in 1 or more doses. It may take 2 or more weeks before you experience the full benefits of the drug. Do not suddenly stop taking trazodone, as it can cause adverse effects such as headache, nausea, and tiredness. Talk to your doctor about gradually reducing your dose.

Side Effects

- Common side effects: agitation, blurry vision, confusion, constipation, dizziness, dry mouth, headache, insomnia, low blood pressure, nausea, and tiredness.

- Less likely side effects: clitoral priapism (a condition in which the clitoris remains erect for a prolonged period), reduced libido, and problems with orgasm.
- Unlikely but serious side effects that should be reported to your health-care provider: abdominal pain, blood in the urine, chest/jaw/left arm pain, fainting, nightmares, ringing in the ears, seizures, shortness of breath, signs of infection (e.g., fever, persistent sore throat), slow/fast/irregular heartbeat, and tremors.
- In young people up to age 25, use of antidepressants such as trazodone may increase the risk of suicidal thinking and behavior. Report worsening depression and/or suicidal thoughts to your health-care provider immediately.

Possible Drug, Supplement, and/or Food Interactions
- Trazodone with MAOIs such as isocarboxazid (Marplan) and phenelzine (Nardil), or with selegiline (Eldepryl), can result in confusion, high blood pressure, and tremor. If you need to switch from trazodone to an MAOI, wait at least 1 week after stopping trazodone before you begin taking the MAOI. After stopping an MAOI, wait 2 weeks before you begin taking trazodone.
- Trazodone can result in increased concentrations of digoxin or phenytoin and an increased risk of side effects.
- Trazodone should not be taken with drugs that have an impact on serotonin activity, such as dextromethorphan, lithium, MAOIs, SSRIs (e.g., citalopram), SNRIs (e.g., duloxetine), Saint-John's-wort, sumatriptan (and other triptans), tricyclic antidepressants, and tryptophan. This combination increases the risk of developing serotonin syndrome, a rare but potentially fatal condition.
- Carbamazepine may reduce blood levels of trazodone.
- Indinavir (Crixivan), ketoconazole (Nizoral), and ritonavir (Norvir) can raise levels of trazodone and increase the risk of side effects.
- Trazodone with psychotropics, such as clozepine, can have a serious impact on cardiovascular function.

Tell Your Doctor
- If you have any allergies and all OTC and prescription medications you are taking, as well as supplements.
- If you have a history of clitoral priapism, a recent heart attack, a personal or family history of bipolar disorder or suicide attempts, heart disease, liver disease, kidney disease, or blood pressure problems.

Of Special Interest to Women

- No adequate studies of trazodone in pregnant women have been done. In animals, trazodone has had negative effects on the developing fetus. Use trazodone during pregnancy only if your health-care provider feels the benefits outweigh the risks.
- Trazodone passes into breast milk. It is generally recommended you not breast-feed while taking trazodone.

Symptoms of Overdose

Breathing difficulties, irregular/slow/rapid heartbeat, seizures, unusual dizziness, unusual drowsiness, and vomiting.

Ustekinumab

Brand Name

Stelara

Available as Generic?

No

Principal Use

Moderate to severe plaque psoriasis for people 18 years and older

About the Drug

Ustekinumab is the first new type of biologic treatment for moderate to severe psoriasis that is potent enough to allow for infrequent dosing. It is approved to treat patients who are candidates for phototherapy or systemic therapy (medications taken by mouth or by injection) and only for plaque psoriasis—not other types of the skin disease.

Ustekinumab works by blocking the immune system molecules interleukin-12 and interleukin-23, which are believed to be abnormally active in the skin and joints of people who have psoriasis. Because ustekinumab is a relatively new drug (FDA approval in 2009), its long-term safety and effectiveness are unknown. Also unknown is whether it may prove useful at some point to treat psoriatic arthritis. Trials to explore this possibility are under way.

In clinical trials, ustekinumab proved very effective in relieving symptoms of moderate to severe psoriasis. During a 12-week trial, about 75% of patients reported at least a 75% improvement in skin psoriasis symptoms, and the improvements continued for most of the patients beyond 1 year. Among patients who had a 75% improvement after 9 months, nearly half of them achieved a 90% improvement at 2.8 years. Because ustekinumab works differently from other biologics for psoriasis, it may be effective for some patients who have not responded to other biologics.

How to Use This Drug

As of 2011, ustekinumab was available only as an injection that must be administered by a medical professional. You will receive 2 initial doses 4 weeks apart and then maintenance doses every 12 weeks thereafter. If you weigh less than 220 pounds, the dose should be 45 mg initially, followed by 45 mg 4 weeks later, then 45 mg every 12 weeks. If you weigh more than 220 pounds, the dose is doubled at each treatment.

Side Effects

- Most common side effects: headache, tiredness, and upper respiratory tract infections.
- Because ustekinumab suppresses the immune system, you may be at greater risk of developing tuberculosis and infections caused by bacteria, viruses, or fungi.
- Ustekinumab may increase the risk of certain types of cancer and cause posterior leukoencephalopathy syndrome, a rare disorder that affects the brain and can cause death. Symptoms include confusion, headache, seizures, and vision problems.

Possible Drug, Supplement, and/or Food Interactions

- Ustekinumab is new to the marketplace; therefore, drug interaction studies have not yet been conducted.
- Because ustekinumab suppresses the immune system, there is potential for interactions if you take other immunosuppressants. For example, ustekinumab may have an indirect impact on how your liver processes cyclosporine and theophylline. Therefore, your health-care provider should monitor you closely and make adjustments to your medications if you are taking ustekinumab along with other immunosuppressants.
- Do not get a live vaccine (e.g., BCG for tuberculosis, nasal seasonal flu) while you are being treated with ustekinumab because you may develop active disease from the live viruses in the vaccine.
- If you get a killed virus vaccine while taking ustekinumab, the vaccine may not prompt an adequate immune response because ustekinumab suppresses your immune system.
- Avoid the BCG vaccine for 1 year before and 1 year after treatment with ustekinumab.
- Ustekinumab may have an indirect effect on how your liver handles warfarin. Therefore, your health-care provider should monitor your drug levels and make adjustments as needed.

Tell Your Doctor
- If you have a history of tuberculosis or any type of cancer, or if you currently have an infection, experience infections that come and go (e.g., cold sores), or have a health condition that impacts the immune system, such as HIV, AIDS, cancer, or diabetes.
- If you plan to receive any vaccinations.
- About any allergies, including food, medications, and additives.
- About all OTC and prescription medications you are taking, as well as supplements.

Of Special Interest to Women
- Ustekinumab suppresses the immune system, which means it increases the risk of serious infections or cancer. Because the average psoriasis patient suffers with the disease for about 50 years, there is the possibility that women will consider the drug for long-term use.
- No evaluations on the impact of ustekinumab during pregnancy have been conducted. Consult your health-care provider about the benefits and risks of using ustekinumab during pregnancy.
- Although the use of ustekinumab during breast-feeding has not been evaluated, proteins similar to ustekinumab are excreted in breast milk, and therefore it is very possible ustekinumab will be excreted as well.

Symptoms of Overdose
Not yet known.

Vitamin D

Brand Names
Various, including but not limited to GNC Vitamin D-3, Lifetime Liquid D_3, Nature's Bounty, Nature Made, Sundown, Weil

Available as Generic?
Yes

Principal Use
Bone health

About the Supplement
Vitamin D is a fat-soluble vitamin that is found naturally in very few foods, although it is added to many foods, including milk and other dairy products. The most natural way to get enough vitamin D is from exposure to sunlight, yet many people fail to get a sufficient amount of vitamin D this way, and so the third option—supplements—is often necessary.

Regardless of how you get your vitamin D, your body must transform it to make it active and usable. The first transformation occurs in the liver, where vitamin D is changed to calcidiol. The second transformation occurs mainly in the kidneys and results in the active form, known as calcitriol.

Vitamin D is especially beneficial for women because it is a critical nutrient for bone strength and density. Without sufficient vitamin D, your bones cannot grow properly, and remodeling by special bone cells cannot take place. Along with calcium, vitamin D can protect against development of osteoporosis, as this vitamin is necessary for calcium absorption. Vitamin D is also involved in neuromuscular and immune system function, reducing inflammation, and regulating cell growth.

When measuring vitamin D levels in the blood, the best indicator is calcidiol. Levels of calcitriol do not typically decline until vitamin D deficiency is severe.

How to Use This Supplement

As a supplement, vitamin D is available in two forms: D_2 (ergocalciferol) and D_3 (cholecalciferol). Experts do not always agree which form provides better nutritional support, but it appears that at high doses, vitamin D_2 is less potent.

According to the Food and Nutrition Board at the Institute of Medicine of the National Academies, women age 19 up to 70 need 600 international units (IUs; or 15 micrograms) of vitamin D per day, while women older than 70 need 800 IU. Many experts, however, believe these daily doses are too low.

The Vitamin D Council, for example, recommends that healthy adults take 5,000 IU daily (pregnant women, 4,000 IU or less) if they do not get adequate exposure to sunlight. The council defines adequate sunlight exposure as regularly receiving 20–30 minutes of midday sun in the late spring, summer, and early fall (use at least SPF8 sunscreen). It is suggested you obtain a calcidiol blood test to make sure your blood levels of vitamin D are between 50 ng/mL and 80 ng/mL (or 125–200 nmol/L) year-round. Your health-care provider will recommend a dose of vitamin D that can help you achieve this goal.

Side Effects

- When taken in recommended doses, vitamin D supplements do not generally cause any side effects. For symptoms associated with long-term use of excessively high doses, see "Symptoms of Overdose" below.

- In some individuals, high doses of vitamin D supplements may cause dry mouth, fatigue, headache, loss of appetite, metallic taste, nausea, sleepiness, and vomiting.

Possible Drug, Supplement, and/or Food Interactions

- Corticosteroid medications such as prednisone can hinder vitamin D metabolism and reduce calcium absorption, which can contribute to bone loss and the development of osteoporosis over the long term.
- Use of the weight-loss drug orlistat and the cholesterol-lowering drug cholestyramine can reduce your ability to absorb vitamin D and other fat-soluble vitamins.
- Phenobarbital and phenytoin increase the metabolism of vitamin D to inactive compounds and reduce calcium absorption.

Tell Your Doctor

- About any allergies you have, and all OTC and prescription medications you are taking, as well as supplements.
- How much sun exposure you get and if you regularly consume foods high in vitamin D (e.g., enriched milk and other dairy products, salmon, sardines).
- If you are experiencing muscle pain, fatigue, symptoms of depression, sleep problems, mood swings, or lowered immunity (e.g., more colds). These are symptoms of a vitamin D deficiency.
- If you have high levels of calcium in your blood, atherosclerosis, sarcoidosis, histoplasmosis, hyperparathyroidism, or lymphoma. Taking the supplements may make these conditions worse or lead to other health problems.

Of Special Interest to Women

- With age, the body gradually loses the ability to utilize vitamin D properly, which in turn reduces calcium absorption rates. This greater risk is especially prevalent in postmenopausal women.
- Recent studies indicate that vitamin D may also help control symptoms of premenstrual syndrome, including irritability, anxiety, and tearfulness. Other studies suggest that vitamin D has a role in relieving depression and helping prevent certain cancers (including breast cancer). Low levels of vitamin D have also been associated with an increased risk of heart disease, stroke, asthma, and high blood pressure.
- Vitamin D is likely to be safe during pregnancy and breast-feeding when taken at levels of 4,000 IU or less. However, discuss vitamin D

supplements with your health-care provider. An overdose in pregnant women can cause mental or physical retardation in infants.

Symptoms of Overdose

An overdose of vitamin D usually occurs over time rather than from a
single excessive dose. The body stores excess vitamin D in fat cells,
where it can reach toxic levels over time. Adults who take 100,000 IU of
vitamin D daily may reach toxic levels within a few months. Signs and
symptoms of vitamin D toxicity include large deposits of phosphate and
calcium in the lungs, heart, and kidneys, where they can cause irreversible organ damage; nausea, vomiting, weight loss, kidney stones, renal
failure, high blood pressure, severe headache, nervousness, excessive
thirst, bone pain, deafness, itchy skin, and heart rhythm irregularities.

Warfarin

Brand Name

Coumadin

Available as Generic?

Yes

Principal Uses

Treatment of blood clots in the lower extremities, atrial fibrillation to
reduce risk of stroke, prevention of blood clot formation after certain
surgeries

About the Drug

Warfarin is an anticoagulant (often referred to as a blood thinner) that is
used to treat blood clots or to prevent new clots from forming in the
body. Warfarin works by decreasing the levels of clotting proteins in the
blood to facilitate smooth blood flow. Treatment and prevention of blood
clots is important to help reduce the risk of heart attack, stroke, deep vein
thrombosis, and pulmonary embolism.

How to Use This Drug

Warfarin is available as tablets and can be taken with or without food.
While you are taking warfarin, your health-care provider will periodically test your blood-clotting time (protime) to avoid excessive thinning
of your blood and an increased risk of bleeding.

Some foods can interact with warfarin (see "Possible Drug, Supplement, and/or Food Interactions" below) and affect how the drug works
in your body. Discuss necessary dietary changes with a knowledgeable
health-care provider if you have any questions.

Side Effects

- Common side effects: abdominal pain, loss of appetite, and nausea.
- Serious side effects: bleeding and gangrene of the skin. Bleeding can occur anywhere in the body.
- Bleeding around the brain can cause severe headache and paralysis.
- Bleeding in the joints can cause swelling and joint pain.
- Bleeding in the gastrointestinal system can cause black tarry stools, coffee ground vomit, fainting, and weakness.
- Bleeding in the kidneys can cause bloody urine and back pain.
- Other side effects of bleeding include bloating, chest pain, diarrhea, easy or unusual bruising, hair loss, painful purple toes, rash, shortness of breath, vision changes, and yellowing of eyes and skin. Report any of these symptoms to your health-care provider immediately.

Possible Drug, Supplement, and/or Food Interactions

- Avoid sudden large increases or decreases in the amount of foods you eat that are high in vitamin K (e.g., broccoli, cauliflower, kale, spinach, and other green leafy vegetables; liver; green tea; and certain vitamin supplements).
- Cranberry juice and other cranberry products may affect how warfarin works. Consult your health-care provider about how much of these products you can safely consume.
- The following drugs can increase warfarin's ability to thin the blood: acetaminophen, amiodarone, aspirin, cimetidine, fluconazole, nonsteroidal anti-inflammatory drugs (e.g., celecoxib, ibuprofen, mefenamic acid), oxandrolone, and quinolone antibiotics (e.g., ciprofloxacin).
- Warfarin should not be taken with imatinib and mifepristone.
- Herbs and natural supplements that have blood-thinning or blood-clotting properties may affect warfarin. These supplements include bromelains, coenzyme Q10, cranberry, danshen, dong quai, fenugreek, garlic, ginkgo biloba, ginseng, goldenseal, and Saint-John's-wort.
- Warfarin may interfere with certain lab test results to measure theophylline. Tell your doctor and lab personnel that you are taking warfarin.
- Use of alcohol while taking warfarin may increase your risk of stomach bleeding.

Tell Your Doctor

- If you have any allergies and all OTC and prescription medications you are taking, as well as supplements.

- If you have a history of alcohol use or abuse, a bleeding disorder, blood disorder, blood vessel disorder, heart failure, liver disease, mental/mood disorder, recent major surgery, thyroid problems, or a vitamin deficiency or absorption problem. Also tell your doctor if any family member has not responded to warfarin treatment.
- If you plan to have surgery, including dental surgery, tell doctor or dentist you are taking warfarin.
- Although the FDA has announced that generic warfarin products can be interchanged, talk to your doctor of pharmacist before you switch to another warfarin product.

Of Special Interest to Women
- Women who have taken warfarin during pregnancy have had children born with birth defects and experienced fetal bleeding. You should not take warfarin if you are pregnant or plan to become pregnant.
- Warfarin does not pass into breast milk. Although there have not been any reports of harm to nursing infants, talk to your doctor before breast-feeding.

Symptoms of Overdose

Black or tarry stools, bleeding gums, dark or pink urine, heavy menstrual bleeding, nosebleeds, and prolonged bleeding.

Zoledronic Acid

Brand Name

Reclast

Available as Generic?

Yes

Principal Use

Postmenopausal osteoporosis

About the Drug

Zoledronic acid is a bisphosphonate, and it works to increase bone density. Because zoledronic acid is given as an intravenous (IV) treatment, it bypasses the digestive system. As of 2011, it was the only intravenous medication for osteoporosis designed to provide 12 full months of protection against fracture, and to offer such protection in the hips, spine, and other bones.

Zoledronic acid is also available as Zometa, and in this formulation it is used to treat high blood calcium levels (hypercalcemia) that may accompany cancer, and with cancer chemotherapy to treat bone problems in cancers that have spread to the bones. It lowers high blood calcium levels by reducing the amount of calcium that leaves the bones and enters the bloodstream.

The information in this entry focuses on Reclast.

How to Use This Drug

Before receiving zoledronic acid, your doctor will likely order a simple blood test to check your blood calcium and kidney function. It is recommended that you drink 2 glasses of fluids, preferably water, a few hours before treatment to help prevent kidney problems. The drug is administered via IV, should not exceed 5 mg, and takes at least 15 minutes to complete the treatment. A treatment can be given by a nurse or doctor and can be administered in a doctor's office or an infusion center. Take calcium and vitamin D daily as directed by your doctor to maintain calcium blood levels.

Side Effects

- Common side effects: flulike symptoms, fever, headache, high blood pressure, and joint and muscle aches. These occur within the first 3 days of treatment and are less likely to occur after the first treatment.
- Unlikely but serious side effects: atrial fibrillation and eye infections such as conjunctivitis or iritis.
- Rare but very serious side effects: acute renal failure, severe jawbone problems (osteonecrosis), and unusual thigh bone fractures.
- Hypersensitivity reactions have been reported and include rare cases of hives, swelling of the lips and eyes, and anaphylactic shock.

Possible Drug, Supplement, and/or Food Interactions

- Zoledronic acid with aminoglycosides may result in a lowering of calcium levels for a prolonged period of time.
- Zoledronic acid with loop diuretics may increase the risk of abnormally low calcium levels.
- Caution should be used when receiving a zoledronic acid injection and taking NSAIDs because of possible liver toxicity.
- Do not use zoledronic acid (Reclast) if you are also receiving the other form of zoledronic acid, Zometa.

Tell Your Doctor

- If you have any allergies and all OTC and prescription medications you are taking, especially diuretics, as well as supplements.
- If you have hypoparathyroidism or malabsorption syndromes (difficulty absorbing minerals in your stomach or intestines), or if you have had thyroid surgery or part of your intestine removed.

- If you have kidney problems or if you have asthma from taking aspirin.
- If you have hypocalcemia (abnormally low calcium levels in your blood). You should not take zoledronic acid injections if you do.

Of Special Interest to Women

- Do not use zoledronic acid if you are pregnant. Tell your physician immediately if you become pregnant while on zoledronic acid treatment, as the drug may harm the fetus.
- Do not use zoledronic acid if you are breast-feeding or plan to breast-feed. It is not known if zoledronic acid passes into breast milk.
- Because there is a risk of severe jawbone problems when taking zoledronic acid, your doctor should examine your mouth before you start treatment. It may also be a good idea to see your dentist before you receive the drug. Practice good oral hygiene (floss!) while using zoledronic acid, as poor dental health, ill-fitting dentures, and tooth extraction may increase your risk of jawbone problems.
- Clinical studies have shown that zoledronic acid can significantly increase bone mineral density at the lumbar spine, total hip, and femoral neck (hip joint). When compared with placebo, zoledronic acid increased bone mineral density 6.7% at the lumbar spine, 6.0% at the total hip, and 5.1% at the femoral neck over 3 years.

Symptoms of Overdose

Significant renal impairment, hypocalcemia (abnormally low calcium levels), hypophosphatemia (abnormally low phosphate levels), and hypomagnesemia (abnormally low magnesium levels).

Zolpidem

Brand Names

Ambien, Ambien CR, Edluar, Zolpimist

Available as Generic?

Yes

Principal Use

Insomnia

About the Drug

Zolpidem is a sedative or hypnotic. Although zolpidem shares some characteristics with the benzodiazepine family of sedatives, it provides much more of a sedative effect and much less of muscle relaxant and antiseizure benefits. These qualities make zolpidem a common prescription for insomnia. Zolpidem improves the ability to fall asleep and to stay asleep longer.

How to Use This Drug

Zolpidem is available as regular tablets, extended-release tablets, and an oral spray (Zolpimist). The typical dose of regular tablets or spray is 10 mg, or 12.5 mg of the extended-release tablets. If you are elderly, your doctor will likely start you at 50% of these doses because older adults have a reduced ability to eliminate zolpidem from the body.

The spray form is absorbed more rapidly by the body because it is absorbed through the membranes in the mouth, and it is a convenient option for anyone who has difficulty swallowing tablets.

Take zolpidem immediately before going to bed and on an empty stomach. Taking zolpidem with food delays the effect of the drug.

Because zolpidem infrequently can cause temporary memory loss, do not take zolpidem unless you have at least 7–8 hours to devote to sleep. For example, do not take it if you want to take a 3-hour nap, as you may wake up with temporary memory problems.

Do not suddenly stop taking zolpidem, especially if you have been taking it regularly at high doses for a long time. You may experience withdrawal symptoms, including flushing, nausea, nervousness, shakiness, stomach cramps, and vomiting.

Side Effects

- Common side effects: diarrhea, dizziness, drowsiness, a "drugged" feeling, dry mouth, headache, and upset stomach.
- Less common side effects: balance problems, confusion, euphoria, insomnia, and vision changes.
- Unlikely but serious side effects that should be reported to your health-care provider immediately: fast/pounding heartbeat, memory loss, mental/mood changes (e.g., new or worsening depression, hallucinations, anxiety, aggression), and unsteadiness.
- Rarely, zolpidem can cause abnormal behaviors such as sleepwalking, sleep-driving, and other activities (eating, preparing food, having sex) while not fully awake and having no memory of these activities. If these events occur (often a partner or other family member notices), contact your health-care provider immediately.

Possible Drug, Supplement, and/or Food Interactions

- Alcohol increases the effect of zolpidem.
- Zolpidem with sodium oxybate can cause very serious interactions.

- Zolpidem increases the effects of other sedatives.
- Itraconazole and ketoconazole may increase the blood concentration of zolpidem.
- Rifampin may reduce the concentration of zolpidem.
- Zolpidem can significantly increase drowsiness when taken with certain antihistamines (e.g., diphenhydramine), antiseizure drugs (carbamazepine), antianxiety drugs (e.g., alprazolam, diazepam), muscle relaxants, narcotic pain relievers (e.g., codeine), and psychiatric medications (e.g., amitriptyline, risperidone, trazodone).

Tell Your Doctor
- If you have any allergies and all OTC and prescription medications you are taking, as well as supplements.
- If you have a history of kidney disease, liver disease, mental/mood problems (e.g., depression), lung or breathing problems, or myasthenia gravis.
- If you have a personal or family history of alcohol and/or other drug use or abuse.

Of Special Interest to Women
- Do not use zolpidem during pregnancy unless your health-care provider decides it is necessary. Infants born to women who have taken sedatives or hypnotic drugs near their delivery time may experience withdrawal symptoms. Consult your health-care provider about the benefits and risks of taking zolpidem during pregnancy.
- Zolpidem is passed into breast milk and may have a negative effect on your infant. Consult with your health-care provider about breastfeeding.

Symptoms of Overdose
Slowed breathing or a deep sleep from which you cannot be awakened.

Bibliography

Introduction

National Center for Health Statistics, Data Brief Number 42, September 2010.

US General Accounting Office. *Report to Congressional Requesters on Women's Health.* July 2001. www.gao.gov/new.items/d01754.pdf.

Chapter 1

Deutch B et al. Menstrual discomfort in Danish women reduced by dietary supplements of omega-3 PUFA and B_{12} (fish oil or seal oil capsules). *Nutr Res* 2000;20:621–631.

Harel Z et al. Supplementation with omega-3 polyunsaturated fatty acids in the management of dysmenorrhea in adolescents. *Am J Obstet Gynecol* Apr 1996;174(4):1335–1338.

Kanadys WM et al. Efficacy and safety of Black cohosh (Actaea/Cimicifuga racemosa) in the treatment of vasomotor symptoms—review of clinical trials. *Ginekol Pol* Apr 2008;79(4):287–296.

McKenna DJ et al. Black cohosh: efficacy, safety, and use in clinical and preclinical applications. *Altern Ther Health Med* May–Jun 2001;7(3):93–100.

Moghadamnia AA et al. Effect of Clupeonella grimmi (anchovy/kilka) fish oil on dysmenorrhoea. *East Mediterr Health J* Apr 2010;16(4):408–413.

Sampalis F et al. Evaluation of the effects of Neptune Krill Oil on the management of premenstrual syndrome and dysmenorrhea. *Altern Med Rev* 2003;8:171–179.

Shams T et al. Efficacy of black cohosh–containing preparations on menopausal symptoms: a meta-analysis. *Altern Ther Health Med* Jan–Feb 2010;16(1):36–44.

Wu CC et al. Metabolism of omega-6 polyunsaturated fatty acids in women with dysmenorrhea. *Asia Pac J Clin Nutr* 2008;17(suppl 1):216–219.

Chapter 2

Baliki MN et al. Beyond feeling: chronic pain hurts the brain, disrupting the default-mode network dynamics. *Journal of Neuroscience* Feb 6 2008;28(6):1398–1403: Also http://health.usnews.com/usnews/health/healthday/080208/chronic-pain-harms-brains-wiring.htm.

Greenspan JD et al. Studying sex and gender differences in pain and analgesia: a consensus report. *Pain* Nov 2007;132(suppl):1:S26–45.

Mogil JS. Sex, gender and pain. *Handbook Clin Neurol* 2006;81:325–341.

Sokka T et al. Women, men, and rheumatoid arthritis: analyses of disease activity, disease characteristics, and treatments in the QUEST-RA study. *Arthritis Res Ther* 2009;11(1):R7.

Tu CH et al. Brain morphological changes associated with cyclic menstrual pain. *Pain* Sep 2010;150(3):462–468.

van Middendorp H et al. The effects of anger and sadness on clinical pain reports and experimentally-induced pain thresholds in women with and without fibromyalgia. *Arthritis Care Res (Hoboken)* Apr 21 2010.

Chapter 3

National Women's Health Information Center. US Dept. of Health and Human Services, Office on Women's Health. WomensHealth.gov/faq/lupus.pdf.

Society for Women's Health Research and the National Women's Health Resource Center. *Autoimmune Diseases in Women,* 2002.

US Department of Health and Human Services. Office on Women's Health. Women's Health Issues: An Overview. Fact sheet, May 2000.

Walsh SJ. Autoimmune diseases: a leading cause of death among young and middle-aged women in the United States. *Am J Pub Health* 2000;90:1463–1465.

Chapter 4

Jackson E et al. *Am Heart J* Feb 2011; DOI: 10.1016/j.ahj.2010.09.030.

Johnson SM et al. Assessment of analysis by gender in the Cochrane Reviews as related to treatment of cardiovascular disease. *J Women's Health* Jun 2003;12(5):449–457.

Lloyd-Jones D et al. Heart Disease and Stroke Statistics—2010 Update: A Report from the American Heart Association Statistics Committee and Stroke Statistics Subcommittee. *Circulation* 2010;121:e1–e170.

Mayo Clinic. www.mayoclinic.com/health/heart-disease/.

Vogel VG et al. Update of the National Surgical Adjuvant Breast and Bowel Project Study of Tamoxifen and Raloxifene (STAR) P-2 trial: preventing breast cancer. *Cancer Prev Res (Phila)* Jun 2010;3(6):696–706.

Chapter 5

National Institute of Mental Health. www.nimh.nih.gov/health/publications/women-and-depression-discovering-hope/what-causes-depression-in-women.shtml.

Whitmer RA et al. Timing of hormone therapy and dementia: the critical window therapy revisited. *Ann Neurol* Jan 2011;69(1):163–169.

Chapter 6

Jamison RN et al. Gender differences in risk factors for aberrant prescription opioid use. *J Pain* Apr 2010;11(4):312–320.

National Institutes of Health. Podcast May 4, 2010, with Dr. Nora Volkow. www.nih.gov/news/health/may2010/od-04.htm.

Petersen EE et al. Prescription medication borrowing and sharing among women of reproductive age. *Journal of Women's Health* Sep 2008;17(7):1073–1080.

Part 2

www.drugs.com/drug-interactions.

Brasky TM et al. Specialty supplements and breast cancer risk in the VITamins And Lifestyle (VITAL) Cohort. *Cancer Epidemiol Biomarkers Prev* Jul 2010;19(7):1696–1708.

Clegg DO et al. Glucosamine, chondroitin sulfate, and the two in combination for painful knee osteoarthritis. *N Engl J Med* Feb 23 2006;354(8):795–808.

Herro-Beaumont G et al. Glucosamine sulfate in the treatment of knee osteoarthritis symptoms: a randomized, double-blind, placebo-controlled study using acetaminophen as a side comparator. *Arthritis Rheum* Feb 2007;56(2):555–567.

IMS Health statistics in *Forbes* article: www.forbes.com/2010/05/11/narcotic-pain killer-vicodin-business-healthcare-popular-drugs.html.

McAlindon TE et al. Glucosamine and chondroitin for treatment of osteoarthritis: a systematic quality assessment and meta-analysis. *JAMA* 2000;283:1469–1475.

Nguyen P et al. A randomized double-blind clinical trial of the chondroitin sulfate and glucosamine hydrochloride on temporomandibular joint disorders: a pilot study. *Cranio* 2001;19:130–139.

Oktem M et al. Black cohosh and fluoxetine in the treatment of postmenopausal symptoms: a prospective, randomized trial. *Adv Ther* Mar–Apr 2007;24(2):448–461.

Plassman BL et al. Prevalence of dementia in the United States: the Aging, Demographics and Memory Study. *Neuroepidemiology* 2007;29:125–132.

Rossini M et al. Evidence of sustained vertebral and nonvertebral antifracture efficacy with ibandronate therapy: a systematic review. *Ther Adv Musculoskelet Dis* Apr 2011;3(2):67–79.

Sawitzke AD et al. The effect of glucosamine and/or chondroitin sulfate on the progression of knee osteoarthritis: a report from the glucosamine/chondroitin arthritis intervention trial. *Arthritis Rheum* Sep 29 2008;58(10):3183–3191.

Seshadri S, Wolf PA. Lifetime risk of stroke and dementia: current concepts, and estimates from the Framingham Study. *Lancet Neurol* Dec 2007;6(12): 1106–1114.

Stopeck AT et al. Denosumab compared with zoledronic acid for the treatment of bone metastases in patients with advanced breast cancer: a randomized, double-blind study. *J Clin Oncol* 2010;28(35):5132–5139.

Resources

American Chronic Pain Association

www.theacpa.org/default.aspx

Information, pain management tools, education, and support for people with chronic pain and their families.

American Heart Association

www.heart.org/HEARTORG

Lots of information on heart disease for everyone.

American Heart Association Go Red for Women

www.goredforwomen.org

A focused effort to fight heart disease in women.

Arthritis Foundation

www.arthritis.org

Much information and research on all types of arthritis.

Centers for Disease Control and Prevention Women's Health

www.cdc.gov/women

The CDC's Web site for women's health issues.

Clinical Trials

http://clinicaltrials.gov

Access to a registry of federally and privately supported clinical trials conducted in the United States and around the world.

Drugs.com

www.drugs.com

Peer-reviewed information on more than 24,000 prescription drugs, over-the-counter medications, and natural products. Also available is a pill identifier, which can help you identify pills, tablets, and capsules.

Endometriosis Foundation of America
www.endofound.org
Provides information, funds research, and helps raise awareness about endometriosis.

HealthyWomen.org
www.healthywomen.org
Covers health topics of interest to women of all ages, from pregnancy to midlife and beyond, nutrition, medical concerns, and exercise.

Lupus Research Foundation
www.lupus.org/newsite/index.html
Information, support, and hope for individuals who suffer with lupus.

National Birth Defects Prevention Study
www.nbdps.org
The Centers for Disease Control and Prevention has a National Birth Defects Prevention Study, which works to identify possible risk factors for birth defects, including the impact of certain medications.

National Institute on Drug Abuse
www.nida.nih.gov/nidahome.html
Information about all types of drugs of abuse, including prescription medications.

National Women's Health Information Center
www.womenshealth.gov
A government Web site that provides the latest information on women's health issues, including current studies, statistics, and information on medical conditions.

Organization of Teratology Information Specialists
www.otispregnancy.org
Provides information to pregnant women about the risks and safety of taking medications during pregnancy and breast-feeding. It also conducts studies of pregnant women who contact them after they have taken certain medications.

PCOS Foundation
www.pcosfoundation.org
A nonprofit that offers support services for teens and women with PCOS.

Physician's Desk Reference
www.pdrhealth.com/drugs/rx/rx-a-z.aspx
A-to-Z listing of prescription drugs and information on diseases and conditions.

Polycystic Ovarian Syndrome Association
www.pcosupport.org
A volunteer organization run by and for women with PCOS and their families.

Pregnancy Registries
www.fda.gov/ScienceResearch/SpecialTopics/WomensHealthResearch/ucm134848.htm
Drug companies sometimes conduct special studies using pregnancy registries, in which they enroll pregnant women who have taken a certain medication. The FDA has a list of pregnancy registries and how to enroll.

PrescriptionDrugAbuse.com
    www.prescription-drug-abuse.org
    Help and information on prescription drug abuse.
WebMD.com
    www.webmd.com/drugs
    A-to-Z listing of prescription drugs and a Pill Identifier.
WomenHeart: The National Coalition for Women with Heart Disease
    www.womenheart.org
    WomenHeart champions prevention and early detection, accurate diagnosis, and
    proper treatment of women's heart disease.
World Endometriosis Research Foundation
    www.endometriosisfoundation.org
    First global charity to foster research in endometriosis to improve knowledge and
    treatments.

Index

About the Author

Deborah Mitchell is a widely published health writer. She is the author or coauthor of more than three dozen books on health topics, including seven books for the Healthy Home Library of St. Martin's Paperbacks (*52 Foods and Supplements for a Healthy Heart; 25 Medical Tests Your Doctor Should Tell You About; A Woman's Guide to Vitamins, Herbs, and Supplements; The Complete Book of Nutritional Healing; The Concise Encyclopedia of Women's Sexual and Reproductive Health; How to Live Well with Early Alzheimer's;* and *The Family Guide to Vitamins, Herbs, and Supplements*), as well as *The Wonder of Probiotics* (coauthored with John R. Taylor, N.D.); *Foods That Combat Aging; Your Ideal Supplement Plan in 3 Easy Steps; Collins Children's Pill Guide;* and *What Your Doctor May Not Tell You About Back Pain* (coauthored with Debra Weiner, M.D.).

About the Consulting Medical Editor

Marjorie Luckey, M.D., is an associate professor of reproductive science at Mount Sinai Medical Center in New York City and medical director of the Osteoporosis and Metabolic Bone Disease Center in Livingston, New Jersey. She holds board certifications in both internal medicine and endocrinology and metabolism. Dr. Luckey is a nationally recognized expert in the field of osteoporosis and metabolic bone disease.